Mrs. Winograd brings excellent skills, sensitivity and experience in writing this book. She is an accomplished and knowledgeable psychotherapist. She has had cancer for which she received curative treatment. This is a wonderful book and will be particularly helpful for the cancer patient and family as well as for those who want to learn about cancer from the informed, intelligent patient perspective. Most particularly, it is upbeat, emphasizing the importance of patient and family becoming knowledgeable about cancer and participating in the decision-making process. She emphasizes that research in new treatments which are promising are becoming increasingly available, offering hope for the individual patient today and the expectation of further progress in the treatment of the disease. She deals in a very sensitive and effective manner with such problems as fear, tumor recurrence, psychosocial, family and financial complexities. In all, it is highly informative and a pleasure to read.

Emil Frei, III, M.D.
Physician-in-Chief, Emeritus
Chief, Division of Cancer Pharmacology
Dana-Farber Cancer Institute
Boston, MA

GET HELP,
GET POSITIVE,
GET WELL

SARAH WINOGRAD

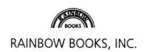

RAINBOW BOOKS, INC.

GET HELP, GET POSITIVE, GET WELL
The Aggressive Approach To Cancer Therapy
Copyright 1992 by Sarah Winograd
Cover Art: Therese Cabell
Interior Design: Marilyn Ratzlaff
Published by Rainbow Books, Inc.
P. O. Box 430
Highland City, FL 33846-0430

Printed in the United States of America.

Price: $16.95

Library of Congress Cataloging-in-Publication Data

Winograd, Sarah, 1928 -
    Get help, get positive, get well : the aggressive approach to
cancer therapy : a resource book / by Sarah Winograd.
        p.   cm.
    Includes bibliographical references.
    ISBN: 0-935834-78-8
    1. Cancer--Popular works.   I. Title.
RC263.W53 . 1991   90-28716
    616.99'4--dc20   CIP

WARNING/DISCLAIMER
    Every effort has been made to make this collection of materials as complete and accurate as possible. Nevertheless, information may change, there may be mistakes, both typographical and in content. Important data may be omitted. Therefore, this book should be used as a general guide only and not as a final source of information.
    Further, all statements made by the author, Sarah Winograd, are based on her own personal research and study; they do not necessarily reflect the beliefs of all health professionals. It should also be noted that in no way is any information contained herein meant to take the place of or to provide any kind of medical advice or treatment, nor does it preclude the need to seek the advice of a physician. Anyone with cancer or any serious disease must see a qualified expert.

DEDICATION

To my dear husband, Seymore, who was always there!

CONTENTS

ACKNOWLEDGMENTS

Now that *Get Help, Get Positive, Get Well* is completed, I find myself back at the beginning to say, "Thank you," to all of those people who helped me achieve my purpose and goal. Writing this book was an enormous job — seven years of long grueling nights, unbelievable highs and painful lows. Had I known in the beginning what was involved, I might never have written the first word. Yet, after I sent copies of the manuscript to some of the cancer patients with whom I work, and, in turn, received their warm appreciation for the encouragement and helpful information, I can truly say that all the blood, sweat and tears were worth it. For each person that this book may help, I am grateful.

Most of all, though, I am grateful to the One Above for giving me the wisdom and ability required to research and write what you will read here. It is with much awe and deep humility that I say, "Thank you, God."

On another level, I want to thank all the patients, their families and friends whose circumstances contributed so much to these pages; I learned all kinds of wondrous things from them. I cherish every tear we shed together; the knowledge I gained from them — their unbelievable courage and strength — is beyond belief, even beyond words.

Meanwhile, countless numbers of people helped me along the way. To name them all would be impossible, but to each and every one of them, "Thank you." Many others who made important contributions to the outcome need to be mentioned. I shall begin at the beginning . . .

My gratitude to my cousin Sybil Goren Henry, who

introduced me to the art of writing, and to Ruth Levine, who read and reread the book and made important suggestions for it from beginning to end, and to Dr. Stephen Miller, Professor, Department of Counseling, School of Education, Barry University, to whom I owe my counseling skills. I deeply appreciate the wise counsel and encouragement I received from Dr. Emil Frei, III, Physician-in-Chief Emeritus and Chief, Division of Cancer Pharmacology, Dana-Farber Cancer Institute; my long-time friend, Milton Eder; our cousin and good friend, author Lawrence Rubin; literary agent Rollene W. Saal; Sharon Schwartz; author Carol Cohan; Rifka Mendelsohn; Bernice and Bill Schwartz; and Harold Kushner, author of *Why Bad Things Happen to Good People*. I am grateful to Dr. Adrian Legaspi and Dr. Bernd-Uwe Sevin of the Sylvester Comprehensive Cancer Center of the University of Miami, and Helen H. Baldwin, M.S., Associate Director, University of Wisconsin Comprehensive Cancer Center, for their careful review of my manuscript, and to Rabbi Levi I. Horowitz, and Dr. Stan R. Cohen, Chairman, Department of Humanities, Southwestern University of Health Sciences, for reading the manuscript and their encouraging remarks. My appreciation to Bob Leavitt for his help and for their patience with my frequent phone calls and the important information they provided, my thanks to Jo Beth Speyer, Director, and Maria Morales, both of National Cancer Institute (NCI) Cancer Information Service for Florida and Georgia; and to Penny Ashwanden, Director of the Division of Communications and Development, Columbia University Comprehensive Cancer Center, Eric Rosenthal, Director of Public Affairs, Fox Chase Cancer Center, as well as the many specialists I mention in my text who gave of their time to explain to me many of the procedures and treatments I write about; and to Dr. Vincent T. DeVita, Jr., when he was Director of the NCI and to the too-many-to-mention directors and department heads of the NCI-designated Comprehensive and Clinical Cancer Centers who were so generous in sending to me the medical material that was crucial to the book.

I am grateful to Cima Starr for her edits of my early chapters, to Roberta Morgan, health writer, for her in-depth critique of my book and her important suggestions; for the careful and helpful editing of the manuscript by Marilyn Bowden, Erica Meyer Rauzin, Susan Hannan, medical editor; and for the painstaking work of the Rainbow Books, Inc.'s staff, namely, Peggy Bryant, Marilyn Ratzlaff, Therese Cabell, and a very special thank you to my publisher Betty Wright and editor Betsy Wright-Lampe for helping me to get it all together, for their unending support and encouragement, wise advice and their gentle guidance.

But I mustn't forget my family, especially Momma. From the beginning she has been one of my staunchest supporters, and my uncle Philip Shaulson for teaching me to persevere in my studies. Then, there's the rest, unfailing with their encouragement. I am grateful to my brother, Morton; my sisters, Shelley and Raynah, and my dear nieces and nephews who eagerly awaited my arrival in New York to read and comment on my new chapters. And for their ongoing support, helpful suggestions and for lighting up my life, I offer my gratitude and love to my son and daughter-in law, Yehuda and Tsirel, their delightful children Moshe, Malka Leah, Yaakov Mordechai, Charna Beila; my son Jeff; and my dear husband, Seymore . . .

Thank you, one and all, and so many more, too. You will remain with me always between the pages of this book and in the warmth of my heart.

TO THE READER

This book is a guide on *how to be an informed patient.* From the quest for an accurate diagnosis to the search for a second opinion to the need for good follow-up care, this is a manual for cancer patients and an empathetic exploration of a patient's stress, fears, anguish and hopes. Its therapeutic nature should help patients develop the skills needed to cope with their disease.

Each case is different; each person is unique. My hope is that this medical, practical, psychological, and philosophical information will be relevant and useful to the reader.

Drawing from my own experiences as a two-time cancer survivor and a psychotherapist (with a speciality in counseling cancer patients and their families), I work through these pages to guide people toward protecting their own best interests.

The book takes you through the maze of cancer treatment options. It tells you how to be a partner in your own survival, how to ask the right questions and get the right information, and how — and why — to find a second opinion at one of the top cancer centers in the country.

Make no mistake, cancer kills. But many more people survive cancer than is commonly believed; it is not a death sentence. Some survive even its deadliest forms. I am living proof. And fighting for your life is worth the effort. This book won't guarantee your survival, but you can take action to increase your odds, and you can learn what being a survivor is all about: not living forever, but living each day to its fullest.

Get Help, Get Positive, Get Well grew out of my own battle with cancer and is, I believe, a useful guide both for cancer patients and for those medical professionals involved in cancer care. Doctors, nurses, social workers, counselors, family members and others will discover tools they can use in dealing with the often devastating emotions that cancer patients experience.

I begin by examining the cancer profile and how I fit it — and I share some of the pitfalls many patients experience, as well as my own. Having cancer involved me in deep soul-searching to discover the wellspring of my life; it forced dynamic changes in personality, the examination and eradication of habits deeply embedded in the comfortable patterns of middle age. It made me re-examine my most intimate relationships, including the one with myself. At times, this was painful, but the results were overwhelmingly positive.

I've been told that this is a necessary book. It is not a Pollyanna, keep-a-stiff-upper-lip approach; it is an aggressive, down-to-earth, honest guide. Because cancer information can be hard to handle, I've focused on being concise and positive, on using simple and practical language, and on delivering the insistent, optimistic message that cancer patients can and *must be* aggressive advocates for their own survival.

When I learned I had cancer, I did not know what to do. Numbing fear gripped me from the first moment. Did I have any choices? Could I make an intelligent decision in my condition?

I had climbed to the summit of my ambitions only to find a fire-breathing dragon on the mountaintop. I didn't know how to fight dragons. I had to ask questions, but first I had to figure out which questions to ask. I had to arm myself. I studied. I prayed. I made mistakes. I stumbled. But slowly I became impressed with what I could accomplish. Eventually, I got to be a pretty good dragon-slayer.

Read this book in any way that works for you: front to back, or dipping into chapters that seem particularly relevant. However, it is particularly important to read the chapters on The Fear Factor, Second Opinion, Cancer Centers, The Cutting Edge, Becoming An Expert, The Patient's Pledge, The Mind/Body Connection, and Nutrition Alert. I have highlighted the end of most chapters with a personal experience that relates to the material within. The anecdotes are relevant and can be of help. They are optional reading.

It is not my intention to tell you what you *have* to do. I merely explore options of what there *is* to do. I invite you to take away whatever part or parts seem right for you and use them to persevere.

The places, people, and case histories mentioned are real; I've protected the patients' privacy by changing their names. I also have streamlined some medical details.

I encourage you to read this book with an open mind, alert to the genuine potential of good health. You can be your own best warrior. You can triumph. While I hope readers will get many messages from this volume, one message is more important than all the others:

There is always reason to hope.

Sarah Winograd
Miami Beach, Florida

PART I

IN THE BEGINNING

Chapter 1

A PERSONAL PRELUDE:
THE IMPACT OF DIAGNOSIS AND
THE JOURNEY TO SURVIVAL

"My cup runneth over."

As I approached the podium to accept my diploma on a bright afternoon at the University of Rhode Island more than 17 years ago, the joyful words of the psalmist rang in my head. A lifelong dream was being fulfilled. Here I was in cap and gown, graduating at the top of my class, with my wonderful husband and our two sons looking on.

For years, I had juggled my college education with the demands of family life, sometimes with a potholder in one hand and a textbook in the other. Now I had made it, and I was vibrant, happy, eager for the future. I didn't know that the new but persistent pain in my throat was signaling a dreaded disease, or that three scant years later I'd be fighting for my life.

No one can be prepared for the diagnosis. It catches you unaware. You may have stocks and bonds, savings and insurance to carry the financial burden of catastrophic illness, but few people have a plan for dealing with disease itself. The idea seems morbid to many. The very word *cancer* is taboo in polite company; we try to sugar coat it by calling it *The Big C*. But there is no sugar-coating. This was the big time. I had to fight to win. And I did. Along the way, I found new tools for recovery, new ways of asking questions and requiring answers, new sources of relief, and new spirituality.

My experience with cancer led me on a long and painful search for the treatment that would save my life. I had to discover a game plan: how to find help, where to go, whom to see, what to ask. What was the best treatment for my disease? Could I rely on my doctor to refer me to the best available care? If not, could I find it for myself? There was so much to learn. First, I learned to be an aggressive patient, and that was a key factor in my survival.

My cancer was diagnosed on October 19, 1976, miles from my Miami home, where we had moved from Rhode Island after returning from our year in Israel. It was vanquished through a tough course of chemotherapy, surgery and radiation, and it recurred 18 months later. Aggressive, experimental chemotherapy defeated it again. Fortunately, I have been well since.

The previous paragraph is deceptively simple. It is the bare outline of a long struggle that ultimately improved the character of my life and taught me lessons that can strengthen yours.

My life was not extraordinary. I grew up in a happy, loving, busy home in Providence, Rhode Island. My mother worked with my father in the family coal and oil business, yet she was always available when we needed her. Momma was our rock; Daddy taught us unconditional love.

Our home was the gathering point for countless friends and relatives. No one got past the kitchen, where good food and stimulating conversation were always being served. It was exciting and rich in warmth, humor and tradition. I was the oldest daughter. Like me, my two younger sisters, Raynah and Shelley, adored and looked up to our older brother, Morton, who teased and protected us.

When I completed public school, I worked as a bookkeeper and office manager. I moved to New York City in search of independence and matrimony, but in 1956 I married a man from my home town. I was 28 (an old maid in those days) when I shocked friends and family by marrying the most sought-after bachelor in our circle, Seymore Winograd. He is one of the kindest men I have ever met.

We started married life in mid-Manhattan, but after two years we returned to Providence. Our sons, Yehuda and Jeffrey, were born within eleven months of each other, and grew up in the warmth of our extended families.

Shortly after graduation from the University of Rhode Island, my family and I were to spend a year in Israel. There, in the center of many of the world's religions, my sons would learn the deepest meaning of their heritage. This dream pushed me through long nights of studying, trying not to think of the housework piling up. It was a punishing schedule. At times, I wanted to chuck everything, scream, or just sleep for a long time. But I kept my frustrations to myself. "Sarah is a very private person," my husband Seymore told people. I was proud of that apparent strength, but it really amounted to an inability to share my feelings, even with the people closest to me. I kept everything festering inside — a classic, cancer-prone personality.

A profile of a typical cancer patient — though none of us is really typical — is a highly charged, self-contained person who needs to be in control, is bent on winning, and is always racing the clock. That was me. A person who appeared highly motivated and successful, but often, inside, had a poor self-image, a smoldering volcano of pent-up emotions and stress.

Dr. Lawrence LeShan's book, *You Can Fight For Your Life*, describes the typical cancer patient. The most prominent trait is a lack of a true sense of self, which is frequently followed by an inability to express anger or resentment. This stems from a poor self-image, leads to overcompensation and ultimately, to hiding behind a *facade of benign goodness*. Anyone who sees these traits in himself or herself would be wise to explore such cancer-prone tendencies with a therapist. I consider this *cancer prevention insurance*. I wasn't that self-aware. It took cancer to get my attention.

I don't remember when I began to feel the constant, nagging pain, like the beginnings of strep throat. Now and then, when in the doctor's office with my sons, or when having a routine annual check-up, I'd mention it. The doctor would peer down my throat and say there was nothing to worry about. And I'd let it go at that. After all, he was the professional, I was busy, and there was no time in my whirlwind life to coddle myself.

Change was in the wind. There was college, my sons' Bar Mitzvahs — marking their approach to manhood — and, finally, our family's beautiful year in Israel. Financial difficulties forced us to return from Israel sooner than planned, and while we were there, my dear father died. I mourned his passing in Israel and, back home in Rhode Island, I mourned him again. After many frustrations and delays with the man who offered to purchase our Rhode Island home, we finally sold it and moved to Miami Beach, a town so different from Providence that it might have been in another country. The pressure was enormous. I see that now; I did not see it then.

Meanwhile, the little problem in my throat worsened. From time to time, I had consulted doctors in Israel and at home. One internist told me, "I don't see anything. Maybe a tranquilizer will help." The unspoken message was that I was acting like a middle-aged-woman hypochondriac. Because of my own insecurities, I bought the put-down.

Another doctor treated me for strep throat. When I developed laryngitis in Miami, an ear, nose and throat specialist put me on antibiotics. That didn't help either. On my next visit, he said that my thyroid was *palpable*.

He ordered a thyroid scan. It was negative, but the pain grew worse. For a week, I felt as if a fist with rough knuckles was pushing up my throat. It was excruciating. Although I was afraid of becoming a nuisance, I summoned all my courage and called the doctor again. I mentally rehearsed a hundred comeback's in anticipation of the receptionist's put-downs. I hurt physically and emotionally.

The receptionist, adept at shielding the doctor, curtly reminded me that my scan results were negative. I got the message: "Don't bother the doctor." I backed down. That was a crucial mistake.

I was being treated like a neurotic woman complaining about imaginary ills. I agonized privately over my fear and the sight of the slowly enlarging lump in the middle of my neck. Today, I would insist on the doctor's opinion. Today, I wouldn't settle for the receptionist's retort. But like many people, I was easily intimidated. I was in awe of doctors. In a country as health-conscious as ours, in a century during which medical research has taken miraculous strides, this is not surprising. Because of the high priority and esteem given their profession, doctors rank second only to clergymen as objects of our veneration. Some would say they've taken over first place. But doctors are people, not deities. They are subject to the same failings that plague the rest of us: vanity, sloppiness, ego. Some are more brilliant than others. It is up to the patient to find the diamonds among the rhinestones.

Today I'm amazed that I gave that receptionist more credibility than my own pain and anxiety. If I had been more assertive, my cancer might have been detected sooner and healed more easily.

Everything changed on a sultry Thursday night. I kept getting up to close the windows and turning on the air-conditioner, as I felt I was suffocating. Every now and then Seymore would get up, open the windows, and turn it off.

"What's the matter with him?" I thought irritably. "Can't he feel this humidity? It's choking me. Either he's crazy or I am."

Friday morning, I woke up choking. Something was pushing through my throat. I now knew that it wasn't the heat. Something was very wrong.

This time, no receptionist could stop me. I demanded to see the doctor that day. He looked in my throat and immediately called in his associate. They told me I needed a biopsy, the removal of a small piece of tissue to examine under a microscope for cancer cells. They would schedule one at the nearest hospital as soon as possible.

They didn't offer me any alternatives.

They didn't tell me if this was the best hospital for my condition.

They didn't tell me what would happen next.

P.S.: I didn't ask.

I was an intelligent adult, a college graduate with a psychology major, yet I asked nothing. I was numb.

I left the doctor's office gripped by a cold fear that sapped my strength; I felt like a zombie. It was late Friday afternoon, close to the time to inaugurate the Sabbath. Nevertheless, on the way home, I stopped at my brother Morton's house and hurriedly told him about my visit to the doctor and my fears. He winced, hugged me, and said, "Bay (his nickname for me), in synagogue tomorrow, I'll have the Rabbi make a prayer for your speedy and complete recovery."

I found comfort in his words. I felt connected to that higher source available to any person who can turn to a personal creed in times of crisis.

I arrived home, quickly finished some preparations, put some money in the charity box, and stopped to offer a fervent prayer that things would be put right for me.

The hardest step was telling my husband. We clung to each other and had only minutes to shed a few tears. The cloudburst that was threatening would have to wait. I struck the match and said the blessing over the lighting of the candles to usher in the Sabbath.

Years of conditioning, habit and self-discipline took over. Jews throughout the world put aside the daily difficulties of life to welcome the Sabbath with peace and joy. The howling inside my head subsided. I was able to quiet the fear, to give myself over to spirituality. The Sabbath was my anchor, my place of rest from the turmoil of the week — and of this dreadful specter. It was my source of strength.

The inbred habit of observance, and the love and comfort of my family carried me through the Sabbath and beyond the initial shock. Then the questions came . . .

What if I didn't have a biopsy?

What if I went elsewhere?

What came next?
What were the odds?
What were the risks?
What was happening to me?

I could hardly bear to look at my sons. I wanted to dance at their weddings, to hold my grandchildren in my arms. I wanted to live. God, how I wanted to live.

That will to live would become my source of strength. At first, I didn't suspect the power of the life force. Yet at that moment, my surge of determination lifted me out of the doldrums where fear had marooned me. It restored my ability to function.

As clarity returned, I called my sister Shelley in New York. I remembered that she knew Dr. Moses Nussbaum, the Chief of Head and Neck Surgery at Beth Israel Hospital in Manhattan. He was an associate of Dr. Max Som, a pioneer in voice box surgery. Since my voice was coming and going, I reasoned that he would be the doctor to see. To my astonishment, Shelley was able to get me an appointment with him three days later. At last, I had found a top-flight specialist willing to see me, and quickly.

When I arrived at Dr. Nussbaum's office in New York, and he examined my throat, his eyelids closed involuntarily for a fraction of a second. "Uh oh, Sarah," that nearly invisible wince told me, "this is big trouble." But his flinch of compassion also conveyed that, for all his eminence, this doctor cared. Relief flooded through me; he knew what was happening and he was up front with me. Struggling for control, I gave myself over to this man's care and to silent prayer.

"No wonder you feel like you're choking," he said. "You have a growth that's encompassing your entire neck."

Finally, there was a reason. I wasn't imagining things. I was very frightened, but in a strange way, also relieved. I'd known at some level that the persistent pain in my throat was serious, yet doctors kept passing me off as a hypochondriac. Here was a doctor who saw what my body had been telling me for a long time. I was not crazy; I was gravely ill.

Dr. Nussbaum took a detailed medical history of the pain in my throat. The thoroughness of his questions raised a few of my own.

Why didn't my former doctors want a history?

Why didn't I insist on giving them one?

Why hadn't I sought a second opinion long ago, as soon as I realized my complaints weren't being carefully tracked.

Through the course of my illness, this question and others haunted me. I wish I'd been my own champion sooner.

Dr. Nussbaum explained that my persistent pain couldn't have been strep throat or any other minor illness. It indicated a precancerous condition. Addressing me as an intelligent partner in fighting my disease, he described my condition and my options in detail. I would need surgery to remove the growth. It would be examined microscopically to determine if it was benign (non-cancerous) or malignant (cancerous).

As frightening as all this was, Dr. Nussbaum's manner and openness about my condition was reassuring. It conveyed a strong message that he valued me as a human being, believed that I could handle my disease and that he would be there for me.

Chapter 2

The Fear Factor:
MAKING FEAR WORK FOR YOU (MUSTERING YOUR ENERGY AGAINST CANCER)

Fear can make you desperate. You can drown in it. Some people can't even acknowledge it. You think, "Help! What's happening to me? What if I'm maimed and disfigured? What if I become a vegetable? What if I go insane from the pain?" Behind all these what-ifs is a host of new fears connected with death. "What will happen to my spouse? Who will raise my children?"

The *what-if* sequence can loop endlessly in your mind, a private horror show. But you will discover that when you switch to positive thoughts, you can drown out the worry and the negative internal voice. You need to know that there are techniques you can use to help yourself, and there are professionals who can help you to overcome fear.

RESPONDING TO FEAR

The experience of fear is universal. For some people, fear takes the form of an incredulous, angry, "Why me?" Others go through denial, sadness, anger, bitterness, the whole gamut of emotions, with such internal thoughts as "I don't think I'll make it," "I can't handle this," or "I guess I'm going to die." Still others fail to recognize the fear or anger at all.

Elisabeth Kübler-Ross, in her work with terminal cancer patients, concluded that people go through five stages when faced with death:

1) denial (behaving as if nothing is wrong) and
   isolation (withdrawing from others)
2) anger (Why me?)
3) bargaining (If You'll let me live, God, I'll be a
   kinder person . . . or I'll give to charity . . .)
4) depression (low, sad and hopeless)
5) acceptance (that death is inevitable)

Further studies have indicated that not all patients go through all five stages. In my work, I have found that fear is behind each stage. Patients who resolve their fear at the beginning of their illness can move directly into a healthy state of acceptance and are in a stronger position to handle their disease in a hopeful state. Hope, like dread, can be self-fulfilling.

Patients who are literally *scared to death* when they hear their diagnosis and who are not helped to resolve their fear, often internalize the diagnosis as a death sentence. This, too, can become a self-fulfilling prophecy.

Some denial is healthy. It provides a mental buffer zone for absorbing shock. But unexamined fear is lethal in the long run. Unless we learn to cope with fear, it can kill us. Fear immobilizes the body by charging it with intolerable levels of stress, pumping it full of adrenaline. This natural physiological response provides an extra rush of energy, the better to react to perceived dangers, but the body can't maintain that outpouring of adrenaline indefinitely. Scientists call it the *fight or flight* response, alluding to the hunted animal's options: battle the enemy or flee. *With cancer, there is no choice but to fight.*

Failing to fight can do you a great deal of harm. In 1983, a research psychologist and cellular biologist, Joan Borysenko, working with other researchers at Harvard

Medical School and Boston's Beth Israel Hospital, observed that passive cancer patients didn't fare as well as their more aggressive counterparts. I suspect this comes into play when people fail to take aggressive action to dispel their fear or anxiety. Adrenaline released by the fear reaction collects and thus creates additional stress, which can have a debilitating effect on the immune system. This may be a factor in the reduced survival rate among the passive patients in the Borysenko study.

LOOK FEAR IN THE EYE

In your fight for life, the energy that fear itself generates can be a powerful force. But first, you have to acknowledge the fear. Only by dealing with fear, only by looking it in the eye and accepting the awesome nature of your illness, can you release the energy it consumes and use it for other purposes, such as fighting back. By acceptance, I don't mean resignation to your fate; I mean full acknowledgment that your cancer is a fact of life and you must fight it.

In my work, I find the fear factor to be one of the most urgent issues that cancer patients need to work through and resolve.

Listlessness, in response to fear, is not unusual in cancer patients. Many people, particularly those conditioned to think negatively, may resign themselves to dying. Although it seems to indicate a lack of interest in life, this stupor is really a failure to face up to internal emotions. Fear over-amps the emotional circuitry, causing a blackout.

Many cancer patients emerge from that initial listlessness trying to grasp some semblance of control. Many talk of putting their affairs in order. "I'm not afraid to die," they claim. But the real message often is, *"I'm too frightened to do anything but die."* The prospect of lingering illness, debilitating pain, diminished reason, and all the other lurid images the fear-infested mind can conjure up are too awful to confront.

Gaining control is necessary in handling fear. As I

have pointed out, controlled, redirected fear can be a useful weapon. Clearly identify the nature of your fears and come to terms with them.

SIGNALS OF STRESS

As you bring the components of fear to the surface, pay attention to the specific physical sensations each one triggers in you. These reactions differ from person to person. When I'm afraid, I feel as if my very essence is coming out of me, right down through my body and out my toes. I seem to be disappearing from myself. Others have described fear as a tightening of the skin, as if their flesh were shrinking around their bones. Some people feel an icy chill right through to the marrow, some a knotting, strangling sensation deep in the abdomen. Fear can cause nausea, cramps, headaches, anger, insomnia, fever, rapid heartbeat, shortness of breath, and more.

Enumerate your body's signals. As you become attuned to your fear symptoms, you will be able to recognize the onset of an attack of fear. This awareness of your body state is one stage of a mind-body therapy called biofeedback. Biofeedback is the use of electronic equipment to indicate when your body is experiencing stress or is in a state of relaxation. Sensors from the equipment attached to a specific area of your body, such as your scalp or your fingertips, cause the machine to give off a signal that indicates your body state. By attending to the signals of the biofeedback equipment, you can be trained through controlled breathing and other techniques to achieve a state of deep relaxation and therefore eliminate the stress.

Familiarizing yourself with the feeling of tension in each muscle will help you zero in on the subtle body changes that signal stress. As you pinpoint your body's characteristic responses to stressful emotions such as fear, anxiety, anger or sadness, you'll be able to identify stress faster and cope with it more effectively. Awareness of a state of tension can also alert you to the cause of the stress. Lydia Temoshok, a researcher at the University of California, San Francisco, performed studies with patients that showed them how the biofeedback machine registered their emotional response even though they themselves were not always aware of it.

COURAGE . . . ANTIDOTE TO FEAR

To overcome your fears, take a good look at your life and identify factors that give you strength. What makes you eager to survive? Perhaps you have things left undone, loved ones who need you, promises to keep, dreams never realized. You might find that an internal repetition based on *when I'm well again* or *when this is over* can block negative, apprehensive thoughts.

Visualize your life after the struggle is over. This technique of developing a positive mindset can control fear and give rise to the energy you need to fight your disease. Focus on the day when you'll walk jauntily down the street, glowing with health. Picture yourself accomplishing something you've always yearned for, but never found the time to do. Find alternatives to giving in to the frightened inner voice that cries, "Please, no, not me." Have courage.

I see courage as an antidote to fear. You need courage, but you already have more than you give yourself credit for. Believe in it; you are courageous. Dig back into your life. Find those moments when you demonstrated courage. You did, you know, even if you don't consider yourself brave.

Maybe you faced a wartime enemy. Perhaps you responded to a crisis with courage for your child's sake. It need not be something big. Perhaps you defended an unpopular classmate in grade school, a small thing in retrospect, but it required deep reserves of courage at the time. The situation doesn't matter. Just remember the intense fear, and how — in one moment of bravery — you harnessed that energy and turned it into strength.

You need that strength now. No matter how much you try to control it, fear returns now and then. That's natural. When you accept that you are afraid, when you look that monster in the eyes, courage is set free. Then you can begin to manage your fear with whatever coping method works best for you.

You can use relaxation techniques such as the one that follows, which was devised in the 1930s by psychologist Edmund Jacobson, to help you manage your fears. This form of progressive relaxation is referred to as the Jacobson Technique.

PROGRESSIVE RELAXATION:
A TENSION-RELAXING TECHNIQUE

Do the following tension-relaxing technique at least two times a day for a week, until you can put yourself right into the relaxed state. Familiarity with this technique will enable you to become more aware of the presence of stress in any part of your body. Soon you will be able to enter a relaxed state at will.

1. First, stand with your feet slightly apart. Let your head drop onto your chest, your shoulders fall forward and your arms and hands hang limply by your sides. If you can't stand, simply relax your body as much as possible.

Next, shake yourself out until you feel loose as a scarecrow flopping in the wind. When you feel completely physically loose, sit comfortably in a chair.

Then, tighten up your eyes as hard as you can, and hold a few seconds. Feel the strain. Then slowly let go. Let the muscles of your eyes relax. Take your time, paying attention to the pulling down sensation as the muscles loosen. Familiarize yourself with what it feels like when those muscles are relaxing.

Now tense your nose. Feel your nostrils all tightened up, then feel them in a relaxed state. Purse your lips tightly. Feel what it's like with your tongue pushed hard against the roof of your mouth, and experience how that differs from the feeling of your tongue in its relaxed state, your lips relaxed.

Clench your jaw. Relax it. Tighten up the back of your neck. Relax it. Repeat this tensing and releasing with every muscle in your head, and then proceed slowly down your entire body — shoulders, arms, forearms, hands, chest, belly, buttocks, thighs, legs, feet, toes. Retain the memory of what the tense, tight state feels like, and remember the pulling down of your muscles and what it feels like for them to be in a relaxed state.

2. When you complete this tension inventory, remain sitting, breathing slowly and deeply. Place one hand on your chest and the other on your abdomen to monitor the movement of your breath. If your chest rises as you inhale, your breathing is too shallow. To correct this, continue drawing in your breath until the hand on your abdomen rises and the hand on your chest remains still. This tells you that you're breathing deeply. Sit quietly a few moments, listening to your body breathe.

3. You can handle stressful feelings more effectively by taking the relaxing and deep breathing a step further. Meditation can greatly enhance these coping mechanisms. One simple and effective form of meditation is repeating a key phrase. Choose a word or a short phrase that evokes what you want to achieve, such as *peace, love,* or *healing.*

After relaxing your body and monitoring your breathing (as described in the first two exercises), keep repeating your word or phrase in your mind as you inhale and exhale. Focus and concentrate on it, until your mind is cleared of other thoughts and impressions. Other thoughts will seep in — that's okay. Just concentrate on your key word to ease them out.

4. The final process to add to this healing technique is visualization. When you are in a relaxed state, listening to your breathing and concentrating on repeating your word or phrase, picture a peaceful scene: a cascading waterfall, a bubbling brook, a beach where you are basking in the sun. In their book, *Getting Well Again,* Stephanie Matthews-Simonton, O. Carl Simonton, M.D., and James L. Creighton advocate visualizing your cancer cells being destroyed.

Relaxation-meditation-visualization, a multifaceted technique, involves your mind, body, senses and thoughts in a relaxing, healing process.

For best results, meditate in this manner for at least 10 or 15 minutes, two or three times a day. I used this technique all through my chemotherapy. I practiced it whenever I felt anxious, depressed, or stressed. I still use it.

Instruction in the technique is usually given working upwards from the feet and ankles. I prefer working from the top of the head downward, involving the senses and other brain functions from the outset.

Once you have taught yourself how to recognize fear and how to put yourself into a relaxed state, you can practice this portable technique any time you begin to feel stress or fear. If you cannot do this alone, work with a therapist who is trained in relaxation and meditation techniques. Most hospital and clinic staffs include such experts. At times when I feel so wilted I think I can't go on, I flop on my bed or on the sofa and go into this relaxation-meditation-visualization routine for 10 to 20 minutes. It always works. Afterward, I feel rested and refreshed, and I have much more energy to go on.

I have found many patients resistant to getting into relaxation and meditation. I think some of that resistance may be due to an image they have of meditation as being connected to a cult, or some type of religious experience. It is unfortunate that some people think this way — obviously the therapeutic effect is possible without having such a connection.

If you can't do this exercise, that's okay. Not everyone can, and that doesn't necessarily mean that they lessen their chances for survival. Hundreds of thousands of people have survived some of the deadliest types of cancer without exploring any alternative modes of therapy. Researchers don't know with certainty what factors or combinations of factors are therapeutic because there are so many variables.

I do suggest that if you can't do this exercise, at least try to become aware of your body's signals when you are under stress. When this happens, stop short for a moment, both physically and emotionally. Tighten up your entire body and relax slowly. Repeat this exercise two or three times, then take a few deep breaths. Finally, pull out one of the positive mental *tapes* you have *recorded,* and consciously work on resolving your fear.

GETTING HELP

If all this eludes you, if your fear is so all-encompassing that you can't face it alone, get help. Sometimes talking to a friend or relative will help. In the beginning, when the brute fact that you have cancer is so hard to accept, the greatest help and understanding can come from a recovered cancer patient, someone who has already passed through the tunnel you are entering.

Today, most clergy have training in counseling. Many public, private and charitable agencies offer counseling as well. Ask your doctor for a referral, call your community's crisis hot line for information, or check your local library for directory listings.

Whatever you do, don't keep all your pain inside. That may be the hardest advice to follow. After all, it is just that kind of behavior — the urge to be self-contained — that seems to predispose some people to developing cancer in the first place. Fight the impulse to withdraw. Look at your reasons for keeping the walls up — fear, worry, denial — and work to triumph over them. You do not have to be alone. To survive, you're going to have to change. Find someone you can trust and reach out. *You're reaching for your life.*

Although many people associate cancer with death, that connection does **not** have to be made. Cancer patients are surviving every day. Thanks to diligent researchers, the odds are getting better all the time.

"There are more people living with cancer today than dying from it," says Dr. Alan C. Sartorelli, Director of the Yale Comprehensive Cancer Center. "Cancer is no longer a death sentence — over half of the patients with cancer are being cured of their disease."

Many people fear that cancer means unabated agony

and pain for months and years, maybe forever. That is not necessarily so. Even patients who eventually succumb often lead active, happy, fulfilling lives right to the end. One-time presidential candidate Hubert Humphrey and actor Yul Brynner were well-publicized examples.

There is pain, yes. But it was never so bad as I had imagined. My most terrifying thought was that the pain would become so severe that I would act like a wild animal, yelling and screaming, out of control. But I didn't; I was able to deal with it.

Modern medicine has wrought wonders in pain control. Doctors have an arsenal of weapons against pain which they can put at your disposal.

You can call on your doctor for reassurance. Beneath that professional exterior lies a human being with a heart. Don't hesitate to say, "I'm frightened. Can you give me an extra minute or two?" The doctor can provide empathic listening, a comforting touch, or real information that addresses your fears. You're entitled to those resources.

A professional who is experienced in dealing with these problems can help you identify and resolve your fears.

When looking for a therapist specializing in cancer counseling, you could do well with a referral from The American Board of Medical Psychotherapists. Kenneth Anchor, Ph.D., the Board's Administrative Officer, reported that their registry showed 15 to 18 percent of the members with a specialty in cancer counseling. Many types of cancer do not go into total remission; patients with these cancers can live for several years or longer, and are categorized as chronically ill. Board-certified professionals have met criteria that qualify them to work with chronically or terminally ill patients. More information on board-certified psychotherapists can be obtained by contacting: The American Board of Medical Psychotherapists, Physician's Park B, 300 25th Avenue, N., Suite 11, Nashville, TN 37203. The telephone number is: (615) 327-2984.

PUT YOURSELF IN CONTROL

You can't control the outcome of your illness or when your end will come. You *can* control the quality of your life, right now. Do everything in your power to make that life as rewarding as possible. *You have courage. Use it.*

Consider what is the worst that can happen. Death is the toughest fear. Talk about whether you want heroic measures taken. What do you want your loved ones to do if you go into a coma or have to be put on life-support machines? What can you do about how you will die if that time comes? What options do you have? Explore some of them, such as *keep me drugged and out of pain* or *try everything, 'til the very end.*

By discussing these difficult matters with your doctors and family, you can make your wishes known. Control has to start somewhere. This exploration — the genesis of control — can give you some peace of mind, whether the contingencies turn out to be necessary or not.

You can control the decisions being made about your life. This makes things easier for you and for those you love. They are eager to serve you, and now they can, by following your instructions. Once you've been heard and acknowledged, you'll feel that a burden has been lifted. The sense of being in control enhances your response to your disease and your ability to fight back.

. . . PERSONAL PERSPECTIVE

I had one week in New York, before the scheduled surgical biopsy, to be with my husband and sons at the home of friends. Surrounded by my family, I struggled for their sake to appear normal. In fact, I wasn't really there. The part of me that walked and talked naturally, behaving as if I were self-contained and hadn't a worry, ran on automatic pilot. Inside, I was shell-shocked, operating almost entirely on a spiritual plane. Driven by enormous need and fear, I prayed fervently and constantly. As with all rituals that are practiced by people of any faith or inclination, it created a

structure. Cancer patients desperately need structure.

After my surgery, I was still in a state of immobilizing fear. My first recollection was of my sister Shelley hovering at the foot of my bed while a prim, white-haired nurse fussed over me. Miracle of miracles, I could speak to her. I still had my voice! I used it, with trepidation, to ask for a mirror. Was I disfigured? I had to know.

I examined my face. My jaw. My neck was swathed in bandages, yes, but my face was not changed. My jaw was intact. I trembled with relief. I was grateful beyond measure.

I didn't ask about the biopsy result. I didn't ask any questions at all. My emotions were too fragile to handle the news. This, too, seems to have been a healthy state of denial, my mind's way of telling me my computer was overloaded and needed a rest.

I felt no pain. In fact, I felt nothing—no energy, no will. Family and friends came and went, expressing their love and concern. I existed in a trance, listless, remote.

Even though my doctor told me in a compassionate manner that the biopsy was positive for cancer, I went into shock. I was always terrified of health problems; I could handle anything else; I took everything in stride. But when it came to illness I would fall apart. You can imagine what the words, "You've got cancer," did to me. My whole world exploded. But who wouldn't be scared? Cancer is something to be scared about. Putting on a brave front can be just another form of denial. I encourage cancer patients to give themselves permission to cry.

All my life, though, it had been very important to me to maintain self-control. I didn't allow anyone to catch a glimpse of my uncertainty, weakness or fear. I kept my emotions on a short leash, rarely letting them out. With hindsight, I know the calm, frozen expression on my face and occasional questions were the programmed reactions of a robot.

As time passed and I got help in dealing with my feelings, I was able to talk with my husband about my fears of being heavily medicated and out of it. Many patients fear being drugged almost as much as the pain. I was one of them.

Talking through my fears helped me make up my mind that if it became necessary, from time to time, I would have to relinquish the control I so desperately wanted to maintain.

This prepared me for the times when it was necessary to give myself over to medication. I let myself go, and found out it was okay to let go of control occasionally. I didn't have to do that often. I learned that all the things we as human beings fear — pain, drugs, not knowing what's ahead — we can gradually learn to handle. We are wonderfully adaptable and we can get used to almost anything.

I continue to experience fear, but I've learned to deal with it. If I discover a small lump or have a new or persistent pain, I'm afraid. I immediately work to overcome that fear. I talk to someone about it, or if there is no one handy, I talk to myself. I remind myself that I'm a survivor; that if there is a problem, I will be able to handle it. I do deep-breathing, relaxation techniques. If the fear persists, I do not procrastinate. I phone my doctor right away and admit, "I'm afraid. I want you to check this out now."

Chapter 3

The Burden Syndrome:

GO AWAY, BUT NEVER LEAVE ME

Cancer patients often retreat into themselves, withdrawing from those around them, even those who love them most. For terminal patients, withdrawal can be a way of coping when death is imminent. But those who are not terminally ill withdraw as well, motivated by an inability to cope or, most often, by fear, particularly fear of abandonment. Like the elderly nursing home patient who stops eating or caring — this withdrawal behavior can stem from the feeling of being abandoned.

SOLVING THE DEPENDENCY-
ABANDONMENT CYCLE
ટે❧

In many instances, patients withdraw for fear of being a burden. They rationalize this by telling themselves that they are trying to shield the family or that they're being stoic; but family members often feel shut out and rejected. As their pain from rejection grows, being with the patient does, in fact, become a burden. Resentment mounts on both sides. The atmosphere becomes strained. I call this the *burden* syndrome.

It's a vicious cycle that feeds first on the patient's

mixed signals: withdrawal, anger and fear. All the patient really wants to say is, "I know I'm hard to put up with most of the time, but bear with me. I love you so much, and it's hard for me to think I have to be a burden to you."

The fear of abandonment — of being too great a burden to bear — is a basic part of the human psyche. It surfaces in moments of extreme stress or terror. Rather than risk being abandoned by our loved ones, we withdraw. We abandon them before they can abandon us. Following this line of reasoning to its pitiful conclusion, perhaps that's why it's not unusual for cancer patients to leave their spouses.

It's important for families to be aware of the dynamics of this syndrome and to be prepared to deal with it. Otherwise, they may feed into the cycle. The patient who can't express fear of being abandoned only wants to be reassured of your love and your genuine willingness to stand by them through this trauma. However obvious you might think your feelings of affection are, verbalize them.

The patient needs to hear, "I love you very much, and it pains me to have you shut me out of your life. It's okay for you to lean on me. That's what my love is all about."

THE CARETAKER BALANCING ACT

Another aspect of the burden syndrome is that sometimes the caretaker does, in fact, see the patient as a burden. This can be extremely difficult. Usually, the caretaker's perception is subconscious and unspoken. Consciously, the caretaker tries to do everything possible to help the patient.

When a caretaker's fear becomes overwhelming, thoughts come to mind such as, "I don't know how I'll manage. How can I take my wife (husband, brother, mother, child) to radiation treatments every day? I'll lose my job. I'll break down. Then who'll take care of everyone? How will I provide for everybody? How can I leave work? How can I do everything?" The more dependent the patient is, the more difficult the situation can be for the caretaker.

Doctors need to be aware of these reactions. They can

help the distraught caretakers examine their feelings to determine if they are making the best medical decisions for the patient, or if they are opting for the physically or financially easiest way out for the caretaker. A useful alternative in these situations is to suggest that the caretaker hire someone to handle chores that can be delegated, such as shopping, housecleaning and running errands. "Meals on Wheels," transportation to and from doctors, hospitals, or treatments can save a caretaker many hours of effort.

Living in Miami Beach, where a large number of retirees reside, I've noticed a phenomenon that seems to be more particular to their age group — seventyish and above. Many of these people are thousands of miles away from their families — some may be homebound or don't have many friends and therefore feel alienated and isolated. These people can easily fall into the "poor-me" syndrome, which extends into the "burden" syndrome. The "poor-me" syndrome expresses itself in several ways. When family members do make contact, the problem sometimes becomes worse. Patients, hoping to keep the family member involved, exaggerate their dependency needs. This perpetuates the burden syndrome, and thus frightens and alienates the family member.

Some family members or caretakers unintentionally send a cancer patient the message that he or she is a burden. They may be so worried, so harassed with all the extra work of taking care of their loved one that their actions may be abrupt; their tone of voice may be sharp because of their weariness. This can convey impatience or irritability to the patient. Body language can do the same. One patient told me, *"The pity I saw in my mother's eyes was the most painful part of my illness."*

When this cycle of inadvertent negative signals gets perpetuated, the patient can easily fall prey to the burden syndrome. An extreme result might be that the patient cooperates and valiantly dies. Most patients don't want to be a burden. They tell themselves, "I don't think my husband (child, parent, friend) really wants to take care of me. It's easier to face death than have him care for me grudgingly, or to face the fact of being sick and unwanted."

The fear of being a burden may be completely unfounded, but patients can fall into the error of letting feelings of guilt and anxiety dominate their thinking so much that they feel worthless and thus unwanted. Their outlook becomes hopeless.

Further research into the burden syndrome is much needed and should consider the possibility of differences in perceptions from one ethnic group to another — and between men and women as well.

THE GOOD DOCTOR

Wise physicians are cautious to avoid falling into a trap that is often set by the adult children of elderly patients. The well-meaning children may want to make all the decisions about their parent's treatment. The physician needs to address information and suggestions *to the patient*, listening to the patient's response and answering the patient's questions. Doctors who learn what each patient wants have the information essential to carrying out their tasks. This approach is particularly critical in cases that are hard-to-treat or that have poor prognoses. When these issues are addressed in a satisfactory manner, it is more likely that the patient will see himself or herself as a partner in medical care rather than as a burden, and thus better prepared to cope with the treatment.

Physicians need to be aware of these emotional factors, especially in elderly patients. Most people, even if elderly and seriously ill, can readily handle decision-making. In fact, if such patients are given understandable information in a gentle manner, they can usually make the best, most appropriate decision for themselves. But, for this to happen, the physician needs to provide patients with enough time to digest the information, absorb the shocking news, and have sufficient opportunity to discuss treatment alternatives and ramifications.

RESOLVING THE SYNDROME
ह

When a patient, working with a competent therapist, can explore all the aspects of *self*, with all its strengths and weaknesses, that person will come to see the weaknesses as part of humanness, not as signs of failure. Once the therapist helps the patient understand this, the final unfolding and understanding can take place. Then the patient can go on to seek fulfillment of his emotional needs — needs that had not been met because they were not recognized.

As a patient begins to feel good about his or her total self, then the patient will have no problem asking for help. It is the patient with a poor self-image who tends to fall prey to the burden syndrome because he or she doesn't feel worthy of having someone dedicated to providing all the help needed.

Unfortunately, negative thinking is too often reinforced by feelings of illness and weakness that come with cancer or any critical or debilitating disease. People who work through these issues (or who have them under control before they become ill) are the ones Dr. Bernie S. Siegel refers to as *exceptional cancer patients*. In his book, *Love, Medicine and Miracles*, he explains that they are the ones who survive longer and who experience a better quality of life, overall, than the patients who see themselves as a burden.

When you feel afraid, reach out, ask for the reassurance you need. Don't shrink from waking your spouse or calling a friend in the wee hours of the night when fears are often magnified, or at the first light of dawn when depression often descends.

You know that you would nurture and support someone you love who had cancer, so realize that now — the shoe is on your foot. Credit those who love you with the same level of care and affection you would offer them. Believe that they are standing by you because they want to, because they love you.

. . . PERSONAL PERSPECTIVE
ได

I struggled mightily with the burden syndrome. With the best of intentions, I withdrew from my family. I thought I was protecting them by keeping my anxiety and pain inside; and I was terrified of becoming a burden. Part of this dynamic was my martyr-type personality—something I see in many of the patients I counsel — that made it difficult for me to let others do things for me. I couldn't discuss with anyone, even my husband, what I was going through. As a result, I added the pain of rejection to the pain Seymore already felt because of his sympathy and fear for me.

Ultimately, my inability to fend for myself led to resentment, and I turned on my husband. I let everything he did for me contribute to my feelings of being a burden. I got so caught up in finding fault with him that I couldn't see I was making myself feel like a burden — the very thing I accused him of doing. No one can make you feel like a burden unless you decide to see yourself as one. If I had been in a healthier state emotionally, I could have verified whether or not Seymore thought I was more than he could handle. And if it had been the case, we could have tried to work out a solution — together!

I was not aware of this dynamic at the time, but I gradually learned how to tell Seymore what I needed from him. I was able to tell him, "Forgive me, Sey, if I get a little mean or irritable from time to time, but I'm so frightened and it's not easy for me to need you to do so much for me. I feel so guilty. I guess it would help if you would just hold me for a moment and tell me it's okay for me to lean on you." This small amount of sharing deepened our relationship.

As I gained insights into my feelings and learned to express them, the emotional effects of the disease were much easier to handle, and I found that I was far more able to help other people work through similar experiences.

PART II

GETTING STARTED

Chapter 4

Second Opinion:
FIRST STEP TO ASSERTIVE TREATMENT

Your diagnosis is the cornerstone on which your subsequent treatment rests. It should be as accurate and thorough as possible. You truly need the best and latest analysis that science has to offer.

So, stop. Take a deep breath. Then run, don't walk, to get a second expert opinion. All patients need a second, and perhaps even a third, opinion after a cancer diagnosis. This is your best investment in survival. The earlier you get treatment, the better your chances will be, but only if it's the right treatment. Be sure that it is.

A diagnosis of cancer dramatically heightens one's sense of vulnerability. This sudden, intimate reminder of mortality underlies much of the fear that a newly diagnosed cancer patient experiences. Yet this is the time to think clearly, and you can. In Chapter 2, I spoke about channeling fear into disease-fighting energy. This chapter lets you know how to put that energy to good use.

When you're swamped with panic and insecurity, you have a tendency to grasp blindly for support. The terrified cancer patient throws himself or herself on the mercy of the physician who has just made the diagnosis. The more helpless you feel, the less you're inclined to question the doctor's judgment. Yet that is exactly what you should do. Tune into the mental message that tells you, "I'm entitled to the best care."

Cancer is usually diagnosed by someone other than an oncologist, a doctor who specializes in treating cancer. General practitioners, family doctors, obstetricians, gynecologists, ear, nose and throat specialists, and dermatologists, among other practitioners, are more likely to be the initial detectors. However competent these physicians may be in their own specialized fields, most are not cancer experts.

Even if your primary physician refers you to a local oncologist, you may still need an additional opinion, unless the local oncologist is particularly expert in your type of cancer. Physicians routinely refer patients to colleagues at their affiliated hospitals. There's no guarantee that a routine referral is the best for your condition, especially if you have a rare or hard-to-treat cancer.

WHERE, WHY AND HOW
TO FIND THE BEST

Seek out an oncologist who has the expertise necessary to treat the disease.

Teaching hospitals are affiliated with medical schools, so their oncology departments are usually excellent, with modern equipment, top doctors and well-trained staff. A teaching hospital also can give you the names of leading specialists in many different cancer treatment fields.

Much of cancer research is conducted at the National Cancer Institute's (NCI) designated Comprehensive Cancer Centers (CCC) and Clinical Cancer Centers, which are excellent resources for expert second opinions. At these centers, you will find the most qualified oncologists with a heavy experience factor in treating the many different types of cancer. NCI, the federal government's national coordinator and watchdog over cancer research, care and treatment, sanctions Comprehensive Cancer Centers (specializing exclusively in cancer) and Clinical Cancer Centers around the country (see Appendix I and Appendix II).

To maintain NCI approval and designation, these centers must pass a rigorous annual examination and must earn a rating of *excellent* in four criteria:

1. The care and treatment of cancer patients in the hospital and as outpatients;
2. Laboratory and animal research leading to the development of treatment plans (protocols) and clinical trials (which evaluate FDA-approved investigational drugs and experimental treatments on patients to establish their effectiveness on different types of cancers) for cancer patients;
3. Professional and lay education;
4. Community outreach, including preventative programs and testing.

Comprehensive Cancer Centers must meet even more stringent requirements than Clinical Cancer Centers. The Cancer Information Service (CIS) toll-free hot line *1-800-4-CANCER* operates out of these centers.

The NCI also funds 56 Community Clinical Oncology Programs (CCOPs) in 30 states. To find the program(s) nearest you, simply call the CIS at *1-800-4-CANCER*. Such programs involve clinics, groups of oncologists or individual hospitals, 270 hospitals, and 2,000 physicians. Through the CCOP system, local oncologists are able to channel their patients to suitable programs in their own communities.

Another function NCI serves is the sponsorship of clinical trial groups in which new treatments are tested. This Clinical Trials Cooperative Group Program (Appendix III) of the NCI creates a link among more than 465 institutions involved in cancer treatment research throughout the United States, in Canada and Europe. The responsibility of these groups is to design and conduct large-scale trials to test the efficacy of the NCI drug development program's new anticancer agents. These clinical trials are conducted by thousands of investigators and are the proving ground for new cancer treatments, including the latest research about the most difficult-to-treat types of cancer.

Locating an expert qualified to handle your case may only require a telephone call to *1-800-4-CANCER.* Tell the operator you would like to make an appointment to see a physician who specializes in your type of cancer. In most cases she'll provide you with information and direct you to the appropriate department.

Your physician or hospital will need to forward your medical records to the doctor who will be examining you for a second opinion. Be sure to include X-rays, any test results and all information from sources other than your physician that might possibly be relevant.

Don't hesitate to ask your doctor for your medical records; legally, they belong to you, not your physician. You paid for them. Your physician may ask you to sign a release, but that's no problem.

I once had a run-in with a doctor who would only supply my records to other physicians, not to me. I wanted to take my records with me when I visited several experts in Boston and New York, but the doctor wouldn't release them to me. I told his secretary I'd sue, but the physician wouldn't budge, and there was no time to make good my threat.

I had to give him the address of each physician I was seeing. And although the records were finally mailed, I got to the consultants before they received any information about my case. Now that most doctors have fax machines, your records are only a phone call away. All you need do is to sign a release form for your records and have them faxed to the doctor's office or cancer center of your choice.

FROM REFERRAL TO CONSULTATION
ક્જ

Just as some physicians will deal only with other physicians, some cancer centers require patients to have a physician's referral. The doctor who made your original diagnosis can set up an appointment for you at cancer centers.

If you are concerned that you might alienate your

physician by asking for a second opinion, just say that your family insists. Generally, any competent doctor will encourage a second, or even a third opinion, especially a creditable one, such as from a CCC. Most physicians would rather not shoulder the responsibility of treating cancer alone when they have the option of expert consultation. In fact, I'd be very leery of any doctor who objected.

If your physician resists your request for a second opinion, take a deep breath and consider his possible motives. Mediocre or incompetent doctors and those with tunnel vision tend to be more overbearing than their numerous professional betters. Don't let yourself be cowed.

Patrick M. McGrady, Jr., co-author of the bestselling *The Pritikin Program For Diet & Exercise*, is director of CANHELP, INC., a worldwide cancer patient information and referral service located at 3111 Paradise Bay Road, Port Ludlow, Washington, 98365-9771. Telephone: (206) 437-2291. He worries about the inexperience and inadequate facilities of community physicians.

"Many of these doctors have learned that they can bury their mistakes," observes McGrady. "It takes courage for a doctor to say: 'I don't know what to do.' and compassion for him to forego the fee and refer to a more competent colleague."

McGrady says he does not wish to frighten patients, but rather to jar them out of a fatalistic complacency. "Reliance upon Good Old Doc Sawbones is a leading cause of cancer mortality," he says. "You must take charge of your treatment and explore your options *before* you start. And you need a buddy to brainstorm with."

He sees an obdurate, panicky wrongheadedness afflicting many patients. He calls it, *The McGrady Syndrome*, named after his father, Pat McGrady, Sr., who had been science editor for the American Cancer Society for 25 years and fell victim to a metastatic bowel cancer in his 71st year. "He knew everybody in the field, all the research, and yet did everything wrong. His diet was loaded with carcinogens; he ignored symptoms for three years; he jumped from one therapy to another, giving none a real chance, and, in the end, fell victim to a cold physician whose bad advice and desultory care ultimately did him in," his son explained. "The patient's fear and confusion are so potent that they can paralyze common sense. Every cancer patient needs the moral support and thinking power of someone close who will hang in there with him or her throughout this experience. It can be family or a friend, a physician or counselor. Someone who really *cares*, though. I will go so far as to say it's almost impossible to hack it alone."

The days of the all-seeing family doctor, the Marcus Welby who has a cure for everything, are long gone if they were ever here. The science of medicine is growing too quickly for any one person to keep up with all the new information. A physician who tried to stay abreast of every advance would have no time to treat patients or to maintain a focus on a medical specialty. The field of cancer research is particularly large, and treatments may change from month to month. That's why you need someone who specializes in your type of cancer.

Remember that people from around the world — royalty and movie stars as well as ordinary citizens — travel to the United States to avail themselves of medical care at our cancer centers, yet our local physicians often don't take advantage of this exceptional resource for their patients. It is amazing that so few Americans even know of their existence.

If you are unable to travel to a Comprehensive Cancer Center, NCI offers another useful service, the Physician's Data Query (PDQ). This has been available to doctors and is now open to the public, too.

PDQ is a computerized information service providing immediate access to the latest cancer research. You can request a PDQ search by calling the CIS at 1-800-4-CAN-CER. It includes a cancer information and treatment file, a directory of more than 12,000 physicians and institutions that provide cancer care, and a file of ongoing experimental treatments around the country. You can get the name of a qualified physician and the most up-to-date information about your type of cancer by using PDQ. More than 400

U.S. cancer specialists act as medical consultants for the service. It is most important to understand that the computer information bank is updated monthly by an editorial board of 21 NCI physicians and an oncology nurse specialist. It is probably the most current source of cancer trials and treatments.

Take the time to use its information, although you'll be bombarded with warnings that speedy treatment is of the essence. These warnings are true. Time is crucial, but barring an emergency, you can usually afford the time it takes to get to the most qualified physician. You've had the condition for some time already. After all, suppose you hadn't been able to see your physician until next week. Just think! *What good is a speedy, incorrect treatment?*

Second opinions are extremely important, so much so that several centers and organizations are prepared to assist patients in obtaining a second opinion, sometimes at no cost or reduced cost, depending on the patient's ability to pay. For example, the Richard A. Bloch Cancer Management Center in Kansas City, Missouri, (see Appendix IV) makes referrals nationwide for all types of cancers. In addition, the Bloch organization provides free consultations by a review board of cancer specialists for patients who live in Kansas and Missouri. During a telephone interview with Richard Bloch, he pointed out that when a patient appears before the panel of experts for a second opinion, none of the doctors who sit on the panel will treat any of the patients they consult with. Thus, the patient can be assured that there is no conflict of interest on the part of the doctor. Mr. Bloch explained, "Just recently our doctors recommended a patient, who needed bone marrow storage, go to M. D. Anderson in Texas (see Appendix I) because that was closest to the patient's home."

If a patient were on the East Coast, they might suggest Dana-Farber Cancer Institute in Massachusetts (see Appendix I), while one living on the West Coast might be referred to the Fred Hutchinson Cancer Research Center in Washington (see Appendix I). There are many

Multidisciplinary Second Opinion Centers (see Appendix IV) throughout the country, which are in part an outgrowth of the Bloch Management Center in Missouri, and were developed to function in a similar manner.

When seeking a second opinion at any one of the Multidisciplinary Second Opinion Centers, a patient may either send medical records to the center for review and be interviewed by a physician who will then review the case with a multidisciplinary panel of specialists and get back to the patient, or in some cases the patient can submit all records for review and later appear before the panel of specialists. At some centers, as at the Bloch Management Center, the patient always appears before the review board. If appropriate, the board will make referrals or recommend further tests or whatever else may be indicated. In some cases, they may say that the treatment plan proposed by the patient's community oncologist is what they would recommend and they may have nothing further to offer.

What is important is that you can be confident that you have a qualified second opinion from a team of recognized cancer specialists. A few of these centers offer the consultation at no charge — others have a consultation fee. Dr. Peter Wiernik, Associate Director of the Albert Einstein College of Medicine and Chairman of the Oncology Department of the Montefiore Medical Center, reports that not only are they a designated Multidisciplinary Second Opinion Center, but patients can call with a request for a brief point of information, and an oncologist will return the call and respond to the query at no charge. The number to call is (212) 920-4826. Many other cancer centers provide similar services. Yale University Comprehensive Cancer Center reports that doctors throughout the world turn to them for pathology reviews to confirm diagnoses. Most Comprehensive Cancer Centers offer such reviews of pathology slides. Your physician need only send your slides and request a review. Through this second opinion channel, patients have access to the latest diagnostic equipment and expertise.

There are many options available, both for referral and for consultation.

A cancer consultation service for physicians and patients is available at no charge at the University of Chicago Cancer Center. To access its toll-free consulting service from out-of-state, call 1-800-482-6917. In Illinois, the number is 1-800-572-3692.

Dial 1-312-684-1400 to access the nation's first 24-hour Brain Tumor Information service hot line. This operates through the University of Chicago Brain Tumor Research Institute and was established by Stephen and Carly Hullcranz whose son, Gregory, died of a rare brain tumor at age fifteen. They hope the service will help others, who like themselves, spend much time and effort to find what there is to do. Patients who call the hot line are given information or if they wish, they can send their medical records, scans, x-rays and whatever else they have to the service for a group of physicians at the University of Chicago to review. A review takes about two weeks. A surgical oncologist or appropriate physician will call the patient and give their recommendation. This is a way of getting a second opinion from a group of qualified experts without the need to travel to the center. For patients with brain tumors who can't afford to get a second opinion, this is a great financial boost. The consultation of these experts is free.

SECURING THE CORRECT CARE
ᢄᔊ

Don't be tempted to rush into treatment without full knowledge of your options. You know the attitude: "I'll try what this doctor suggests, and if it doesn't work, I'll look for somebody else." This sounds logical, but it's a bad idea. As Richard Bloch, cancer survivor and founder of the Cancer Management Center in Kansas City, points out, *"Cancer is a very serious disease that grows geometrically. If not treated properly the first time, there is often no second time."*

Be sure you have the illness, and the form of illness, your doctor says you have, in the place he or she says you have it.

You have no margin for error. After getting the correct diagnosis, the second most important factor is getting the best treatment the first time around. You don't want to end up six months into the process with complications stemming from a faulty or incomplete diagnosis or treatment.

When, or if, your physician's diagnosis is verified, consider your options carefully before you begin treatment. Patients who are not familiar with cancer don't realize that through the course of a cancer treatment many choices may be available. Medicine is not the exact science we imagine it to be. Frequently, there's more than one way to achieve the same result. However, each doctor has a specialty and a preference.

When there is a choice, a surgeon, for example, will often opt for surgery, an effective treatment in many instances. That doesn't mean it's the *only* possible course, but you won't know unless you ask.

Many physicians have tunnel vision, seeing nothing but their own specialty. Physicians need to have some degree of tunnel vision, just to keep abreast of the latest in their specific fields. But each physician must also keep the total picture in mind. So must the patient. Never stop asking questions.

More is at stake than the loss of precious time. Many common treatment methods, such as chemotherapy and radiation, unfortunately can damage your immune system, possibly rendering you ineligible for experimental treatments. You don't want to discover a promising innovative approach for your hard-to-treat cancer only to learn that because of your previous treatment your body cannot tolerate any further chemotherapy.

If you have a rare or hard-to-treat cancer, clinical trials that test new drugs or therapies on human volunteers may be underway. Use the NCI's resources to find out. If you identify a clinical trial in your type of cancer, your next step is to learn if you are eligible. Trial guidelines — *protocols* — are often limited to patients who meet certain medical criteria. A trial protocol may only accept patients with functioning kidneys, or with lungs that work to a specific capacity. Some trials require patients who have never had chemotherapy or radiation; in other cases, trial guidelines mandate patients who have had no previous treatment at all. *If you get rushed into treatment, you may be closing doors behind you!*

Perhaps some new advance could make all the difference. Modern medicine offers many tests and procedures to pinpoint the nature and stage of advancement of various types of cancer. If there isn't anything that might help, you'll find out quickly enough. If there is, be ready to seize the lifeline.

Find out which research facilities or cancer centers are making advances in treating your type of cancer. The chapters that follow will help you answer these questions.

If you don't live near a cancer center — or near one that specializes in your type of illness — it's probably worthwhile to travel, if you can. If you are unable to travel to a distant cancer center, you can check the Multidisciplinary Second Opinion Centers closest to you. Avoiding outdated, inappropriate or ineffective treatment is worth the time and effort.

Once you've gotten a consultation and decided on a treatment plan, you can always decide to be treated by your local oncologist who can follow-through on the recommendations. But only go to a physician who has your complete confidence and faith. If you have any reservations, no matter how silly they may seem to you, think twice. Cancer is a serious disease; you're fighting for your life. Everyone on your team should be a fellow warrior in your battle.

SELECTING A COMMUNITY ONCOLOGIST

If you decide to receive care from an oncologist in your community, there are obvious reasons for choosing this option: inability to travel, an uncomplicated cancer that doesn't require special treatment, or a desire to have your community oncologist whom you trust and are familiar with follow the treatment plan recommended by a specialist at a cancer center.

What are you looking for? You want someone who is competent, caring and totally up-to-date. Perhaps my experience offers a checklist you can use.

I interviewed Dr. Marc C. Saltzman, an oncologist in private practice, and was impressed with what he had to say. Here are some of the points he made:

* How to tell a patient he has cancer is a key issue.
* How much the patient wants to know is determined by careful listening.
* Patients living with cancer symptoms generally sense or even know what is going on in their bodies.
* Patients who are better informed do better medically.
* Most of the time patients can participate and can assist themselves more than others expect.
* Give patients choices but not answers — and time to make decisions.
* Consultation with another specialist for a second opinion is often recommended.
* It's helpful to work with a psychotherapist, who is trained to counsel patients in making decisions about their treatment.

If you are unable to or don't choose to elect any of these options, there are many hospitals throughout the country whose cancer programs are reviewed and analyzed by the Commission on Cancer of the American College of Surgeons. To be approved by the Commission, a hospital program has to meet stringent criteria. Since there are over 1,000 of these programs, to find the hospital nearest you, write or call the Cancer Department, American College of Surgeons, 55 East Erie Street, Chicago, Illinois 60611; telephone: (312) 664-4050, or call CIS.

Seeking a second opinion is not a new or unusual idea in medicine, where professional consultations are the norm. Today, more and more insurance companies and

Medicare require a second opinion before they'll under-write certain types of surgery. *You should be as cautious with your life as they are with their money.*

Patients with advanced cancer, especially those whose physicians have already told them that nothing can be done, may feel that this information comes too late for them. On the contrary, a second opinion from a top-notch cancer center is especially crucial in these cases. Many cancer centers specialize in innovative treatments of aggressive cancers with success rates far above the norm. A cancer that was impossible to treat even a year ago may be controllable today.

Even treatments that buy time are valuable. *The possibility of someone somewhere finding a cure for your type of cancer is no longer slim.* Just holding on for a while could mean you're still around to benefit from the next new treatment.

Be your own staunch advocate. Don't be shy about demanding the best. You aren't as helpless as you feel. Taking an active part in your treatment, especially in the beginning when you have more options than you will later, can make a big difference in your odds of surviving, and in the quality of your life as a survivor.

Finding the right treatment, the right physician, and the right medical facility are the most critical steps you can take toward a cancer-free life.

... PERSONAL PERSPECTIVE
ಒ

When my local oncologist diagnosed a return of my malignancy, he set me up to start aggressive chemotherapy within a week. I did not know the urgency of seeking a second opinion. Like most cancer patients, I didn't even know of the existence of Comprehensive Cancer Centers.

I was very scared, so I phoned Rabbi Levi I. Horowitz in Boston for guidance and a blessing. I knew he was an internationally recognized lay expert on the kinds of medical specialists and treatment centers in the Boston area.

When I talked to him, I told him of my doctor's plans, and asked for his blessing. "Sarah," the Rabbi said, "I'd like you to come up here with Seymore. You'll stay at my home, and I want you to see Dr. Emil Frei, III. He's the Director and Physician-In-Chief of the Dana-Farber Cancer Institute, one of the foremost cancer treatment centers in the country. He's also a professor of medicine at Harvard Medical School."

I was relieved and ecstatic. It was as if the rabbi had lifted a great burden off my shoulders. I had the utmost confidence in his recommendation. But I worried about telling my local doctor. Whatever happened in Boston, I lived in Miami. I'd probably need him eventually. I didn't want to upset him.

Nervously, I explained when I reached my doctor that my rabbi had insisted that I go to Boston for a consultation at the Dana-Farber Cancer Institute. The physician said he couldn't think of a better place to go.

What a comfort it was to hear this doctor agreeing rather than trying to intimidate me! And his non-threatening manner made it natural and easy for me to return to his office when I decided to continue my treatment back home in Miami.

A nice benefit of this crash course in looking out for yourself is the potential for personal growth in assertiveness and self-confidence, a maturation that can improve all other areas of your life, from shopping in the supermarket, to your job, to your close relationships. Whatever the outcome, your life can be enriched.

Chapter 5

CANCER CENTERS:
PERSONAL ACCESS TO
THE BEST IN THE BUSINESS

The special status of cancer centers offers many advantages for patients. First, and most crucial, is the access to the latest research and treatment methods, which are tested at these centers. It is important for you to be familiar with this resource. Had I not been treated at a CCC, I would have been robbed of the opportunity to have high-dose methotrexate (an anticancer agent) — a treatment that was not available to me from my community oncologist.

As you select a follow-up facility, be aware that some hospitals not designated by the NCI as Comprehensive Cancer Centers use the phrase *comprehensive cancer center* in their titles. Many are fine facilities, but they are not NCI-approved centers. Be sure you know your hospital's credentials.

In this chapter, you will be given some examples of the types of special expertise, special equipment, and special research available at these NCI-sponsored centers.

FINDING CLINICAL TRIALS

The NCI has various channels you can use to find out

about trials that pertain specifically to your illness. First you should understand that a clinical trial is a test of a new drug or therapy in a highly controlled environment. In such an environment, patients in clinical trials can receive experimental treatments before such therapies become generally available.

Clinical trials are broken down into categories or phases, representing different levels of research. A *Phase I* trial is the first time a new drug or procedure is applied to human beings after completion of laboratory and animal studies. Since the side effects of new drugs are largely unknown, only patients for whom no other course of treatment exists are accepted into such trials.

When researchers are satisfied that they have found the highest safe dosage and the best way to administer the treatment, *Phase II* tests targeting various types of cancer can begin. If results are promising, *Phase III* — comparing the new treatment to existing standard methods — starts. If the new treatment proves more effective, it reaches *Phase IV*: recognition as the new standard treatment, alone or in combination with other drugs, surgery or radiation.

If you are a candidate for a clinical trial, find out which phase the treatment being tested is in. This can influence your decision to participate. Patients give signed consent and may withdraw at any time.

If you decide to participate and then withdraw, your doctors will discuss other possible treatments with you. If you don't benefit from the treatment, doctors may take you out of the trial and suggest another course of action.

In fact, if you're not benefiting, you'll probably be removed from the trial even if doctors can't suggest another course of action. No one is kept in a clinical trial just so that results can be observed. The patient's improvement is the first priority. If eventual trial results show that one method tested is clearly more effective, all patients in the trial who might benefit receive the superior treatment.

More than two thousand clinical trials may be under way across the country at any given time. With this staggering volume of tests, any attempt to report all the trials available nationwide would be bewildering and counter-productive. However, knowing the range of available trials should persuade you to learn more about new approaches that might help if you are told you need a clinical trial.

Much is being done on the research and experimental end of cancer. If the subject seems heavy to you, you're right. This is heavy stuff, but so is cancer. And if you have it, you want the latest, best treatment available.

Cancer centers also offer more than research and unique treatments. Objective language can't begin to describe the compassionate care these centers offer. They are innovative patient care institutions as well. Patients benefit from access to clinical trial programs, but they also benefit from expert nursing care and from the cancer centers' team approach to treatment.

GETTING CENTERED:
HOW YOU BENEFIT
FROM INNOVATIVE CARE

Oncologists (cancer specialists), surgeons, radiation therapists (doctors who specialize in treating disease by means of radiation), pathologists (doctors who study abnormal conditions of all tissues), psychologists and other specialists review the patient's case as a team. At many centers, this team approach extends to research as well. For instance, teamwork among pharmacologists, biochemists, toxicologists (scientists who study the effects of poisons on the body), and chemists keeps Yale University at the forefront of drug research. The Drug Development Program at the Lineberger Cancer Research Center at the University of North Carolina in Chapel Hill links researchers with physicians to tailor drug therapies to individual patients.

From the cancer patient's point of view, the high caliber of care offered by a team approach is a valuable resource. At the University of Chicago Cancer Research Center, for example, some 1,100 patients are seen in more than 30 multidisciplinary clinics and in-patient programs where diagnosis, treatment and research are combined. The cancer treatment team there, and at other centers, includes nurses trained in oncology. Their special training results in a high level of nursing care because oncology nurses recognize subtle changes in a patient's body, warning signs that might go unnoticed in a less-concentrated setting.

In addition to assigning each patient a primary physician, many Comprehensive Cancer Centers employ a primary care nursing system. Each patient has a single nurse who is responsible for his or her patient's care for the duration of his hospital stay. The medical advantages of such consistency of care are obvious, but it's a psychological plus, too. It's reassuring to know there is a nurse nearby who is on top of your case.

Having a primary care nurse helps ensure that an outpatient's progress is closely monitored from visit to visit, and that any setbacks are carefully noted. When a patient's oncology nurse thinks something is important and brings it to the doctor's attention, that report is likely to carry more weight than the patient's word alone.

If you have a problem or a question while being treated at most Comprehensive Cancer Centers, you may call your center oncologist any time. Most centers give patients an emergency number to call after 5:00 p.m. and on weekends. In my experience, someone calls you back as soon as possible.

At Memorial Sloan-Kettering, nurses on the Supportive Care Team of the Pain Service provide pain management to patients at home and are available for telephone consultation around the clock. Nurses in the Adult Day Hospital are also available by telephone 24 hours a day, seven days a week. I think it's fantastic that a patient can get reassurance at any hour.

The advantages of cancer centers extend beyond state-of-the-art medical care. Trained nurses, counselors and lay volunteers work in programs that nurture the mind and emotions, as well as the body. For instance, USC has a course in clothing design for mastectomy patients to help recovering women cope with the nitty-gritty details of normal life. Students learn to design swim wear, sundresses, or sleeveless nightgowns so women who have undergone mastectomies (breast removal) can wear those outfits and feel comfortable in them.

Dana-Farber developed a program to train recovered cancer patients in *peer counseling* — in giving encouragement to hospitalized cancer patients. Recruitment was done by inviting former cancer patients who were interested in volunteering for a support group for hospitalized cancer patients. They were given some basic training and were connected with hospitalized cancer patients to interact with them in a positive manner.

Little extras help patients and their families deal with the emotional strain of cancer. In Boston, my husband and I took advantage of Dana-Farber's complimentary passes to visit some of the city's historical attractions and to enjoy the respite offered by the city's cultural events.

Centers also offer support groups and facilities for family members. The all-important ingredient of attitude is bolstered in every way. The Babies Hospital at the Columbia-Presbyterian Medical Center also has facilities for mothers who wish to stay with children undergoing bone marrow transplants. If your child needs such treatment, be sure to inquire about the possibility of sleep-over arrangements at your center. The University of Rochester Clinical Cancer Center has designed its facilities around the concept of presenting a positive and supportive approach to patients and their families. Duke University is well known for its innovative approach to the emotional side of cancer patients and their families.

The NYU Medical Center trains its health-care professionals to meet the special non-medical needs of cancer patients and to promote positive attitudes in other staff members. Medical students are taught how to deal with cancer emotionally as well as medically, and the curriculum is particularly strong in the behavioral aspects and difficulties involved in cancer care.

Memorial Sloan-Kettering established the world's first psycho-oncology program, designed to help patients handle the pressures of cancer and its treatments. Through this approach, patients are assisted in dealing with problems of attitude and adjustment as an integral part of the healing process.

Georgetown University Medical Center reports that its home-care program for terminal and pre-terminal patients is the oldest in the country. The center provides free medical, social and nursing care; medical equipment and supplies; and medication. This allows terminal cancer patients who so desire to be cared for with dignity in the loving environment of their family home. The Mayo CCC has a tricounty hospice program on a similar scale. The counselors and volunteers receive special training in the nuances of cancer counseling.

Using Memorial Sloan-Kettering's Pain Service methods, USC researchers reported a 90-percent improvement in their patients' ability to control pain and nausea after chemotherapy. Many centers have developed their own innovations in pain relief and that information is shared within the cancer community so you can expect assistance in this area at all the cancer centers. To get help with the emotional aspects of pain, you can call or write the American Academy of Pain Management (see Appendix V). According to Richard Weiner, Ph.D., Executive Director, they have a national registry of board-certified pain practitioners who can be found in every state. They are the largest society of pain management professionals in the United States. If you request a referral, their registry lists the professionals by specialty as well as by geographical area. Other associations that provide information to professionals on medications, pain management, referral societies, and conduct outreach programs, support groups and teach coping skills to those in pain can be found in Appendix V.

Memorial Sloan-Kettering's innovative Pediatric Day Hospital — the first of its kind in the country — enables young patients to lead normal lives during the treatment. Today, 85 percent of Sloan-Kettering's pediatric patients are treated in the day hospital setting.

Following the success of the Pediatric Day Hospital, Memorial Sloan-Kettering started the Adult Day Hospital as an alternative to in-patient treatments for those patients who need nursing care but do not require overnight hospitalization. Patients receive treatment at the hospital from 8:00 a.m. to 6:00 p.m. and then return home. To further strengthen the link between home and hospital, an Adult Day Hospital nurse is available by telephone, all day, every day. This cost-effective treatment approach (which eliminates the expensive in-patient hospital stay that requires more nursing care and other routine in-patient services) has been replicated at other cancer centers.

The Ambulatory Oncology Center at Columbia-Presbyterian in New York City has provided outpatient cancer care to all patients in need — regardless of their ability to pay — since it opened in 1983. More than 27,000 patient visits a year qualify the center as a major facility for cancer care in the Manhattan area. In addition to getting their treatment in a comfortable, friendly atmosphere, patients benefit from support groups to help them deal with the emotional ramifications of living with cancer, and a social worker aids patients with medical coverage, home health services, and transportation to and from the center. How I would have treasured a service such as this when I spent six weeks in a hotel in Manhattan while I traveled for daily radiation therapy. The biggest ordeal each day was to get back and forth to the hospital for treatment.

LEARNING ABOUT SPECIAL
EQUIPMENT AND PROCEDURES
ა

Cancer centers' state-of-the-art equipment could be particularly important to you. For instance, the University of Alabama at Birmingham and the Yale and Columbia-Presbyterian Cancer Centers reported having the country's first, costly DNA (deoxyribonucleic acid, the substance present in the nuclei found in the center of cells that makes up the genetic program which directs all the activities of each cell) sequencers, which are now more generally available. Molecular biologists use this equipment to study the structure of DNA, which harbors many of the mysteries of cancer. Information garnered with this equipment has led to new discoveries about how a normal cell becomes cancerous (the basis of researchers' attempts to destroy cancerous cells).

Ohio State University CCC reported specially equipped operating rooms to permit *intraoperative radiation*. These specifically designed operating rooms have radiation equipment that can deliver radiation directly to the site of the tumor while the patient is on the operating table and the tumor is exposed. Though this procedure is available at many medical centers, it, as well as others, were developed and initiated at Comprehensive and Clinical Cancer Centers. The NCI has been a leader in developing modifications in this approach.

CT-GUIDED BIOPSY

Comprehensive and clinical centers often have sophisticated diagnostic equipment before it is in widespread use. One example of this is CT (computed tomography)-guided biopsy which can sometimes be used in cases that might otherwise require exploratory surgery. In CT-guided biopsy, a CAT scan is taken while the patient is in the radiology suite under sterile conditions. Using the scan to pinpoint the tumor, the surgeon can biopsy the exact site without having to conduct extensive surgery to find it.

One advantage of the CT over the X-ray machine which gives a two-dimensional picture is that a three-dimensional picture is produced by the CT.

Nearly all cancer centers have magnetic resonance imaging (MRI) diagnostic equipment. The MRI scanner is not an X-ray but can often be used instead of X-rays or other scanners. The MRI does not expose you to harmful radiation, as an X-ray does. This is a highly detailed diagnostic device that portrays the body's soft, internal tissue, giving safer and sharper images. Memorial Sloan-Kettering boasts

New York's highest powered MRI, as well as highly trained physicians who interpret the tests' results.

Detroit's CCC, Harper-Grace Hospital, Wayne State University, houses one of only twelve MRI Research and Imaging Centers planned for the United States. The MRI center includes three units, with use divided between clinical and research applications.

The eyes that read the test results are far more important than the machinery, so even though there may be MRI equipment at your community hospital, if you need MRI, consider which doctors or specialists will interpret the results of your scan. Your local hospital's doctors may be thoroughly qualified, but cancer center doctors are experts. They see only cancer cases and are so immersed in the study of cancer that they seem to develop almost a sixth sense in detecting its presence.

The University of Texas M. D. Anderson Cancer Center is one of the world's largest. In one year alone, it served more than 31,000 inpatients and 348,548 outpatients. With numbers like that, you can imagine the amount of experience the doctors have. The staff includes 700 nurses and 225 residents and fellows, an impressively high concentration of professionals and scientists with expertise.

DISCOVERING NEW TREATMENT PLANS

Cancer centers cannot guarantee a cure any more than a local oncologist can, but they can offer the benefit of the most up-to-date research. Cancer specialists working to conquer this disease work interactively. They go to national and international meetings and symposia. They read and contribute to professional journals, where they communicate their successes and their failures.

Since the Food and Drug Administration (FDA) maintains strict standards and won't authorize a new cancer drug or treatment for general use until exacting criteria are satisfied, there is a gap between the discovery of a new treatment and its availability to a doctor in a general hospital.

This time, which is spent in clinical trials and exhaustive paperwork, may be time a cancer patient doesn't have.

You will read about bone marrow transplantation in Chapter 6. The Fred Hutchinson Cancer Research Center in Seattle, a pioneer in bone marrow transplantation has performed more bone marrow procedures than any other institution in the world. Its doctors have successfully used this method to treat many different types of cancer of the blood and the lymph system.

Another treatment innovation that was initiated at Comprehensive and Clinical Cancer Centers is intraperitoneal instillation, a way to administer chemotherapy directly into the abdominal cavity, thus minimizing damage to healthy organs. Instead of giving chemotherapy traditionally (by mouth or by injection into the bloodstream or muscles), administration of chemotherapy directly to the site of the tumor allows doctors to give larger doses of anti-cancer agents directly to the site of the tumor.

Also on the cutting edge of treatment, you may remember the excitement generated by Dr. Steven A. Rosenberg and his colleagues in their experimental immunotherapy, interleukin-2 (IL-2), which was developed at the NCI in the mid-1980s. Studies about this new drug at NCI's Surgery Branch in Bethesda, Maryland, and the NCI-Frederick Cancer Research Facility in Frederick, Maryland, showed promising results for many types of cancers. Immunotherapy is designed to use substances to strengthen and support the body's immune system so it can be used as a defense against the cancer that has invaded the body. (More about this in Chapter 6.)

Promising new treatments go through a rigorous testing process. Cancer drugs under study are classified into *Group A, B* or *C* programs. *Group A* drugs are in studies that evaluate the safety and effectiveness of the anti-cancer agent. *Group B* drug studies establish the potential of the anti-cancer agent against specific cancers. *Group C* drugs have already demonstrated adequate anti-cancer results to warrant FDA and NCI approval for more extensive but controlled distribution.

As a result of further testing at additional centers, reports indicated that modified *Group C* programs of these IL-2 therapies were the best available treatment for advanced kidney cancer or advanced melanoma (malignant skin cancer), the most aggressive of skin cancers. IL-2 is a substance in the body that researchers used to treat white blood cells to activate their potential to produce immune system cells (LAK — lymphokine-activated killer cells) that react against cancer cells. By August, 1989, however, the use of IL-2 for melanoma had become controversial. It is not recommended for every patient. Change is rapid in the field of cancer research. That is why you always need to consult with an oncologist who is current on the results of the latest clinical research trials.

CANCER CENTERS:
IT'S NEVER TOO LATE
३☙

These are some of the many reasons I urge you to think of Comprehensive Cancer Centers and Clinical Cancer Centers as first resorts — not last resorts. Although I urge you to check into the many advantages that a cancer center offers, not every case of cancer must be treated at a comprehensive center. Space limitations alone make that impossible. Yet, too many cancer patients wind up at a Comprehensive Cancer Center only after every other avenue has been closed.

Even if you are not treated at a cancer center, contacting a center for information can save you crucial time; centers have programs to provide the knowledge you need. For instance, the University of Southern California and the Jonsson CCC at UCLA coordinate the Cancer Management Network, a consortium of 27 Southern California hospitals involved in clinical trials and experimental treatment. One phone call to this network gets you the most up-to-date information on 27 hospitals in one region.

NCI's designated Northern California Clinical Cancer Program (NCCP) is another one-call source for information about an entire region's cancer-fighting resources. The NCCP, which extends into northern Nevada, includes four medical schools, several major universities, and some 250 hospitals, research institutions and private anti-cancer organizations. NCCP operates four community outreach programs with supervised clinical trials. When time is of the essence, sources like this are lifesavers.

Information is not the only outreach effort that comprehensive cancer centers make. Treatment outreach is available as well. Eric Rosenthal, Director of Public Affairs at Fox Chase Cancer Center, reports a network program that has affiliations with community and larger hospitals, some as far away as Harrisburg, Pennsylvania, whereby patients unable to travel to Philadephia can now have access to clinical trials as well as the expertise at Fox Chase. To locate physicians and a hospital close to your home, contact the Fox Chase Network and Research Affiliates Program at (215) 728-3830. If they are willing to work with a comprehensive cancer center, doctors can gain access to treatments that are not generally available to the public.

As you read in Chapter 4, it is unfortunate when initial treatment methods of chemotherapy or radiation injure the patient's immune system to the extent that the patient is no longer a candidate for experimental or very aggressive treatment. Heartaches like this might be avoided by consulting doctors at a research-oriented cancer center as soon after diagnosis as possible. Nonetheless, it is never too late to seek out the best treatment, the most hopeful path.

... PERSONAL PERSPECTIVES
ಶ್ಠಿ

When I was at Dana-Farber Cancer Institute in Boston, I felt like I was joining a small, self-contained community rather than entering a hospital. The atmosphere was friendly and upbeat. Children play on a large carousel in the lobby. A cheerful volunteer pushes a cart with a gaily-striped awning, offering hot chocolate with marshmallows, coffee, tea and crackers.

This relaxed, positive and caring atmosphere is one of Dana-Farber's many strengths, but it is not unique to that center; a similar pleasant environment is found in many cancer centers. It makes it easier for the patient to face returning for frequent treatments.

When my lymphoma, the cancer that originated in my lymph system, returned, it was diagnosed by my doctor in Miami. I got a second opinion at Dana-Farber, where I was put on high-dose methotrexate in addition to an aggressive chemotherapy protocol. At that time, use of methotrexate was still experimental for my type of malignancy. After three treatments, I came home to Miami to continue chemotherapy with my local oncologist. Access to the high-dose methotrexate of Dana-Farber's clinical trials was possible because of my local physician's willingness to handle the necessary reporting, to follow the trial protocols (experimental trial treatment procedures), and to remain in communication with my oncologist at Dana-Farber.

I'm grateful I had the kind of community oncologist who didn't feel threatened by working in conjunction with a Comprehensive Cancer Center.

Chapter 6

The Cutting Edge:
INNOVATIVE APPROACHES TO DIAGNOSIS, PROGNOSIS AND TREATMENT

The information in this chapter is highly technical. I've made an effort to explain this material in as simple language as possible. Since this chapter may not be easy reading, I suggest you go through it once lightly. It is *not* important for you to understand all the dynamics of these technologies. What *is* important is that you are aware that they *exist*. Bear in mind, though, that not every procedure or test mentioned is used for every cancer. If you think something applies to your situation, go back and reread that section. If you still think it's a way to go, you need to explore and discuss this with your medical oncologist.

If your oncologist appears to be knowledgeable about what you ask and gives you a valid answer as to whether the procedure in question is or is not applicable in your case and he or she can answer quite readily and with apparent familiarity any further questions you might have, you can probably rest assured with the recommendation. If you have any qualms whatsoever about the advice you receive it is never, as I stress, inappropriate to seek a second opinion.

Because these new techniques are frequently expensive and not always covered by insurance, often hard to locate, and sometimes controversial, not all physicians routinely order them. Be sure to select a qualified oncologist who keeps abreast of research and the cutting edge of cancer treatment. Today's new techniques are often tomorrow's practices.

GETTING THE DIAGNOSIS

TUMOR MARKERS:
SITE OF ORIGIN

Different types of tumors produce different chemical substances as they grow. Physicians analyze these chemical *markers* to learn about a tumor's nature and growth. These tumor markers help doctors determine the type of cancer a patient has. This knowledge is essential because, as was said, the type of cancer determines the choice of treatment. Researchers also use these technological advances to detect the spread of cancer. Some of these can alert doctors to a tumor's potential to metastasize (spread).

LYMPHOMA TEST

DNA Gene Rearrangement Analysis is a sophisticated medical test for the diagnosis and recurrence of leukemia and lymphoma. Dr. Walter Voigt, Director of the Diagnostic Molecular Biology Laboratory at the University of Miami School of Medicine, reported their Department of Pathology was the first to introduce to the State of Florida the DNA Gene Rearrangement Analysis. He stressed its importance in diagnosing lymphoma, a kind of cancer that originates in lymphocytes (a type of white blood cell), accurately and properly, since it is not always easy to tell if a particular tumor is a lymphoma as many nonmalignant conditions may mimic lymphomas.

Because lymphoma is difficult to diagnose, this test is unique in its accuracy in diagnosing the disease. It is able also to accurately identify malignant lymphomas from benign lesions. Another unique aspect of this test is that it provides a *fingerprint* of a given tumor, which makes it possible to track a lymphoma when it is in remission. Thus both response to therapy can be documented and a recurrence can be picked up at a very early stage. Dr. Voigt stated that the present detective system is adequate for most lymphomas but researchers use DNA Gene Rearrangement Analysis to provide advanced technological information as a guide in the use of innovative treatments.

THE SPECT CAMERA

SPECT (Single Photon Emission Computed Tomographic) imaging is a technique that has effected considerable improvements in diagnostic performance and in nuclear medicine. I first learned of it when I read of a team of researchers from Technion's Faculty of Medicine and Rambam Medical Center's Nuclear Medicine Department, both in Israel, who during the 1980s were at work on a way to predict which tumors can be treated by chemotherapy. And they are trying to pinpoint, once the tumors have been identified, the effective doses of specific drugs needed to affect a particular tumor. This is being done by making a chemotherapy drug radioactive. The drug can then be tracked using a special SPECT camera manufactured in Israel by Elscint, Inc. that can pick up the amount of the chemotherapy that has reached the site of the tumor.

The highly sophisticated SPECT camera is expensive, but it has proved its value. Since training and experience are very valuable with any new technology, it is important to learn who is operating the camera and who is interpreting the information. The SPECT camera requires that technologists possess technical excellence.

Though it is like the CAT scan, SPECT imaging can be more sensitive. When SPECT imaging is used to gather cancer information, monoclonal antibodies — those which can attach themselves to specific cancer cells — are loaded with a radioactive tracer and directed to the tumor. With gamma technology, beeps are emitted to indicate how much of the material has reached the site of the tumor.

I queried several community hospitals and one medical center had a GENESYS gamma camera. General Electric (GE) and other American manufacturers market comparable gamma cameras. Though each manufacturer develops his own unique SPECT characteristics, all systems are based on general basic principals.

PROGNOSTIC TESTS

FLOW CYTOMETRY

Flow cytometry is a highly sophisticated technique that has many capabilities, one of which is the ability to provide important information to cancer researchers about a cell's DNA, the element present in every cell that directs all of the cell's activities. Through the measurement and study of the DNA structure in cells by the use of flow cytometry, those tumors that are likely to spread and to become aggressive can be identified. Flow cytometry is used to determine the possible course and outcome of solid-tumors such as cancers of the breast, ovary, prostate, colon, and bladder as well as certain cancers of the lung.

TUMOR MARKERS
FOR PROGNOSIS

A flow cytometry DNA Index which measures the amount of DNA in a cell takes no more than 30 minutes when fresh tissue is received by a laboratory qualified to do this testing. A DNA Ploidy Analysis of the flow cytometry results which can be done in two days indicates the degree of variation of the DNA pattern in the cells. This technology makes it easier to identify the cancer being investigated as to the stage of development. For example, this can be helpful in identifying breast cancer tumors — even when they are detected early and are very small — that have a potential to become aggressive and spread.

Tumor markers aside from DNA Index and Ploidy Analyses that are being used to predict the probable outcome of a breast cancer are estrogen receptors and level of cathepsin D. Though these markers have not been consistently accurate and at times conflict with other more established predictive indicators, they provide additional information that can be helpful in making a decision on how to proceed in the treatment of breast cancer. Many physicians are reluctant to use some of these markers as guides to treatment planning because they are not always consistent. Most breast cancer patients, on the other hand, whom I have worked with want these new types of analyses to be performed and are angry with their physicians when they were not told of these options. A typical remark from a patient was: "I want everything possible to be done that can help me make a more informed decision."

CHEMOSENSITIVITY ASSAY TESTING: WHY YOU NEED TO ASK

Chemosensitivity assay testing is a procedure that helps predetermine which treatments might be effective for your cancer. Such information is obviously important in your decision-making process.

This technique allows scientists to study the reactions of a patient's tumor cells in the laboratory to a number of anti-cancer agents. These drugs are tested *in vitro* (in a test tube) outside the patient's body on human cells that have been preserved — and in some cases grown — from biopsied tissue from the patient's tumor. The fact that a chemotherapy works in the laboratory does not guarantee that it will work *in vivo* (in the patient's body), yet the assay can spare the patient the debilitating process of being treated with several different chemotherapies to see which ones are going to fail. With this testing, researchers are now investigating the possibility of using an assay to indicate the highest dosage (of whatever drug is found potentially effective) needed to destroy a patient's cancerous cells.

Larry Weisenthal, M.D., Ph.D., is the originator of the Weisenthal DiSC Assay. This is the assay used for hematologic cancers (of the blood and blood-making tissues), such as leukemias and lymphomas. Dr. Weisenthal is at Weisenthal-Dill Cancer Resource Group, 15201 Springdale St., Huntington Beach, California 92649, (714) 894-0011, where he applies his DiSC Assay and others, and tailors them to accommodate each patient's tumor type.

The Weisenthal DiSC Assay is also used at Oncotech Inc., 1791 Kaiser Avenue, Irvine, California 92714. The telephone number is 1-800-662-6832. The company also has a KERN Assay (developed by David H. Kern, Ph.D.) for solid tumors (tumors which form a mass or growth), such as those of the breast, ovaries, bladder, colon and prostate. The assay can be completed in about a week.

Another chemosensitivity assay test, the fluorescent cytoprint assay developed by Dr. M. Boris Rotman at Brown University's School of Medicine, is available from Analytical Biosystems Corporation, 55 Access Road, Warwick, Rhode Island 02886-1056. The telephone number is 1-800-262-6520.

The fluorescent cytoprint assay can effectively test about 16 different chemotherapeutic agents for their effectiveness against a specific patient's solid tumor and the assay can be done in eight to ten days.

Upon request, these laboratories will send your doctor supplies with instructions on how to submit tissue from a biopsy of your tumor. That tissue is sent to the company via overnight delivery. If a full biopsy is not possible, they may be able to conduct assay testing with a small tissue sample. But the tissue *must* be a fresh sample; it *must* be preserved in a specific medium; and it *must* be handled as the lab directs, so if you are going to have a biopsy, discuss this in full *beforehand* with your oncologist or surgeon. These assays are not cheap and are not always covered by all insurance carriers. Yet, many patients feel that the information is important and are willing to pay for the assay. This advance is very exciting because positive effects of both single and combination drugs can be shown quickly.

Assay testing is no panacea — as its innovators would be the first to tell you. Yet if your tissue is resistant to, say, 16 tested chemotherapeutic drugs, you may want to discuss with your physician if you have a choice of other treatment options. If so, you might want to consider other options first.

If you are looking for an investigational trial, chemosensitivity testing can also help your oncologist and you make a specific selection. If, in assay testing, your tumor responds to a particular chemotherapy, it might make sense to enter a trial using that anti-cancer agent.

Assay testing is done at many cancer centers and some, like the Sylvester CCC University of Miami Medical School, have their own ATP Chemosensitivity Assay (ATP-CSA) which was developed by Bernd-Uwe Sevin, M.D., Ph.D., and other researchers of the Gynecologic Oncology Department.

Most tumors are biopsied by general surgeons, many of whom unfortunately do not know about this type of assay testing. That is why, unless you require drastic emergency surgery, you should not hurry into a biopsy or surgery until you have studied all the options. The use of the chemosensitivity assay is affected by whether or not chemotherapy might be a way to go.

TREATMENTS

STEREOTACTIC BRAIN SURGERY

Stereotactic gamma knife surgery is a treatment method for brain tumors that are inaccessible either by surgery or by radiation therapy. During this procedure the patient's head is immobilized. This allows the gamma knife to rotate around the head while directing the full force of the carefully calculated radiation dose to the tumor tissue. It avoids doing damage to healthy parts of the head and neck, and allows for a much higher dose of radiation to be directed to the tumor.

The Presbyterian University Hospital in Pittsburgh installed the first unit in August 1987. Now many hospitals and cancer centers throughout the country have also acquired it. While researching information for a patient I was counseling, I discovered that Baptist Hospital in South Miami had this costly and highly sophisticated equipment.

I also found that the University of Miami School of Medicine/Jackson Memorial Medical Center had designed and built a halo device that attaches to the patient's head to restrict movement and, like the gamma knife, allows for treatment of deep brain tumors with high-dose X-rays.

Without using the prohibitively expensive gamma knife, innovative researchers at the Columbia-Presbyterian Medical Center in New York City developed an intricate computer program to perform the stereotactic surgery which pinpoints the brain tumor and delivers a sharp high-intensity beam of radiation in much the same way as the gamma knife. For further information about these pioneering techniques or clinical trials being conducted through the Brain Tumor Cooperative Group, call 1-800-4-CANCER.

BONE MARROW TRANSPLANTATION

One new technique that clinicians at cancer centers are turning to more and more often is bone marrow transplantation (BMT). For lay purposes, this treatment can be catalogued into three main categories: *autologous* (involving the patient's own cells), *allogeneic* (involving a healthy donor's cells), and *syngeneic* (which is quite rare as it would have to be a graft only between two genetically identical twins).

Autologous BMT begins with the removal of a portion of the patient's own bone marrow after treatment with chemotherapy and/or radiation (to try to destroy the malignant tumor or tumors).

The patient's treated bone marrow cells — which are now free of cancer — are re-injected to encourage normal white blood cell production. White blood cells, also called leucocytes, the foot soldiers of the immune system, lead the system's attack on diseased cells. The hope is that a strong, healthy immune system can destroy any stray cancerous cells that escaped the radiation or chemotherapy.

In allogeneic BMT, a healthy donor's cells are injected into the patient (after the patient receives radiation or chemotherapy to destroy the tumor) to encourage production of normal, healthy white blood cells. In both types of BMT, the patient is isolated in an antiseptic environment. This protection from bacteria and viruses is necessary because the immune system is so depleted. The hospital room is kept germ-free; anyone who enters dons a sterilized gown, mask and gloves. Anything that is brought into the room — food, clothing, linens — is sterilized.

In a procedure pioneered at Dana-Farber Cancer Institute in 1983, donor cells are washed in monoclonal antibodies to lower the risk of rejection, a syndrome known as graft-versus-host disease (GVHD). In GVHD, the newly transplanted marrow/immune system (particularly the T-cell component) identifies the recipient (patient) as foreign and launches an attack against the patient. Symptoms can range from mild to severe (skin rashes, jaundice, diarrhea and liver disease) and may even result in death. Early and prolonged treatment with the group of drugs known as corticosteroids, along with other medications, is effective in treating most patients who experience GVHD. (See Chapter 9 for more information on BMT.)

HYPERTHERMIA

Several cancer centers are testing whole body, regional and local hyperthermia, or heat therapy, in which a patient's tissue temperatures are raised to a very high degree. These approaches spur a decrease in tumor size. Whole body hyperthermia involves increasing the entire body temperature, excluding the head; regional hyperthermia addresses a specific area of the body; local hyperthermia focuses directly at the cancer site.

Whole body hyperthermia reaches cancer cells far from the original tumor site and gives doctors an additional weapon when metastasis (spread of the cancer cells) has occurred.

Hyperthermia is often used in conjunction with chemotherapy and radiation as it appears to increase the effectiveness of these treatments.

It is also being used with increasing frequency in investigational trials on cancers of the brain, breast, colon (colorectal), pancreas, head and neck.

The American Cancer Society funded a trial at the University of Arizona in which brain tumors were treated with hyperthermia in conjunction with radiation. This university launched joint research into hyperthermia with the University of El Valle in Cali, Columbia, as early as 1972, where it was discovered that tumors often responded better to radiation after they were heated. Research in hyperthermia, hyperthermia in combination with radiation, and other hyperthermia protocols (programs) are being used to treat many types of cancers at many other cancer centers.

When I called to verify a clinical trial in hyperthermia at the University of Arizona, Thomas C. Cepas, Ph.D., a physicist with the Department of Radiation Oncology, told me about their very comprehensive program. In their treatment planning, research is closely integrated with clinical applications. From the first patient they treated in 1977 with a grant from NCI, they have developed their treatment to include local, regional, and whole body applications. Physicists are responsible for certain technical aspects of radiation such as the accuracy and safety of the equipment to ensure that the actual prescribed dosage is being properly delivered to the patient.

Dr. Cepas explained that most comprehensive, clinical or university cancer centers performing hyperthermia belong to the North American Hyperthermia Group. This is a research society whose purpose is to develop basic research and clinical applications of hyperthermia for cancer therapy. Membership in this group allows for academic research within a professional community. International organizations, including the European Society of Hyperthermic Oncology and the Japanese Society of

Hyperthermic Oncology work with the North American group. International congresses are held approximately every four years. The address for the North American Hyperthermia Group is Laura F. Jones, American College of Radiology, 1891 Preston White Drive, Reston, Virginia 22901. The telephone number is (703) 648-8900.

Not all hospitals and medical centers are equipped to provide hyperthermia. Yet, as early as the spring of 1985, Dr. Robert Heller, Chief of the Department of Radiation, at Cedars Medical Center in Miami, reported the use of local and regional hyperthermia at Cedars.

A few years later, Baptist Hospital of South Miami began local and regional hyperthermia treatments in their facility. Similarly, the University of Miami CCC reported that they, too, were equipped to administer local or regional hyperthermia. Don't limit yourself when you are researching special equipment or a treatment plan. Although I recommend that you investigate a Comprehensive or Clinical Cancer Center first, you never know what is in your own backyard.

Because hyperthermia involves an extremely complicated and delicate procedure, it is advisable to go to a center with a great deal of experience in this form of treatment and a large success rate in your particular type of cancer. For example, American International Hospital in Zion, Illinois, reports that they have conducted approximately 1,300 successful whole body procedures in more than 13 years — the largest number performed in the world. They use whole body hyperthermia on all tumors other than those of the brain, those involving the spinal cord or leukemia. The hospital also has an extensive program in local hyperthermia to treat easily accessible tumors such as those of the breast, head and neck, colon, Hodgkin's disease, lymphomas, and melanomas. For information about their program, you can call 1-800-322-9183 to speak to an Oncology Information Specialist.

Two examples in addition to American International Hospital and the University of Arizona (mentioned earlier) of other physicians performing whole body hyperthermia are at the University of Texas Medical School at Houston and the University of Wisconsin Comprehensive Clinical Cancer Center at Madison. Dr. Joan M. C. Bull, at (713) 797-3588 in Houston, has an 11-year record in treating patients with melanomas, colorectal and breast cancers, and Dr. H. Ian Robins, in Madison, reports that he has performed over 700 whole body hyperthermia treatments for breast and lung cancers, lymphoma and melanoma. Dr. Robins' telephone number is (608) 263-1416.

Washington University in St. Louis, Missouri, has one of the longest records in the use of local and regional hyperthermia. They are also doing deep hyperthermia. They have much experience with hyperthermia for superficial tumors, those on the surface of the body, and in places that can be reached through natural openings such as the bladder or cervix. Inquiries can be directed to the Hyperthermia Nurse, Radiation Oncology, Mallinckrodt Institute of Radiology at Washington University. The telephone number is (314) 362-2034.

Another facility with special expertise in this area is Stanford University in Stanford, California, where Dr. Daniel Kapp is Director of the Clinical Hyperthermia program. His telephone number is (415) 723-6939. Some of the cancers treated are those of the head and neck, the chest wall, skin, and deep-seated tumors primarily in the pelvis including the gynecological system, colorectal, bladder and prostate.

Dr. Alexander Marchosky, in Chesterfield, Missouri, has been conducting local hyperthermia for brain tumors since 1985. Patients come to him from all over the world. The location, size and grade of the tumor determines the treatability with hyperthermia — patients can send recent scans and medical notes, and Dr. Marchosky will review them at no charge to discover if they are candidates for treatment, or he will recommend options that can be discussed with the patients' oncologists. Patients can get more information by calling Dr. Marchosky at (314) 878-2888, leave a phone number and the name of a contact person, and he will return the call.

BIOLOGICAL MODIFIERS

Biotherapy, or immunotherapy, is recognized as a fourth treatment approach in treating cancer. It can include the use of interleukin 2 (IL-2), tumor-derived lymphocytes (TDL), lymphokine activated killer (LAK) cells, tumor necrosis factor (TNF), interferon, and monoclonal antibodies. These biotherapies are designed to stimulate and direct the body's own immune system to attack cancer cells.

In 1984, Dr. Robert Oldham, who developed the National Cancer Institute's Biological Response Modifiers Program in 1980, founded the Biological Therapy Institute (BTI), a nonprofit medical research and treatment facility that offers biological protocols on an individualized basis to cancer patients who are not eligible for state-of-the-art or experimental trials elsewhere. Their address is P.O. Box 1700, Hospital Drive, Franklin, Tennessee 37065-1700. The telephone number is (615)-790-7535.

The BTI works closely with Cancer Therapeutics, Inc. (CTI), a laboratory research company, to develop innovative treatment plans for the specific needs of each cancer patient. The approach, once it is determined, is discussed with the patient, who is directly involved in the decision-making. Some patients receive conventional treatment (surgery, chemotherapy, radiotherapy) when appropriate, coupled with the biological therapies or whatever custom-tailored approach that is developed for them.

Adjacent to the BTI is the Williamson Medical Center, which serves as the Institute's in-patient hospital facility. The oncology unit has 19 private rooms, each with a sleeper-sofa for the convenience of a family member who may want to stay overnight. Also available for patients and their families is a well-equipped kitchen and a washer/dryer. Because the institute recognizes the emotional needs of cancer patients, it allows patients on the oncology unit to have visitors around the clock. Patients who require extended hospitalization are permitted to go on short outings. Nutritional, emotional, spiritual, and community support, all are components of services available to patients and their families at the medical center.

One very ill cancer patient who was treated success-fully by an institute-designed protocol after he was told he was not a suitable candidate for an NCI trial explained: "When you think there's something that can be tried, being turned down is probably one of the most devastating things that can happen." In government trials, you are not se-lected unless you meet all the criteria of the exact type of cancer being researched. Through BTI, you are accepted if it is determined that you can tolerate the treatment. You will also need to show that you can afford to pay for it, as most insurance companies will not reimburse for the treatment as biotherapy is still considered in experimental stages. Hospital charges are covered by insurance.

Although it is operating in the private sector, BTI won't admit patients who are beyond hope. In fact, staff physicians encourage patients to look into government or other subsidized programs before they incur the expense of the BTI program.

Another innovator is Dr. James Neidhart, Director of the University of New Mexico Cancer Center, 9000 Camino de Salud N.E., Albuquerque, New Mexico 87131. The telephone number is (505) 277-2151. The center re-ports complete remissions in more than 50 percent of women with advanced breast cancers. Dr. Neidhart's ag-gressive form of chemotherapy is many times higher than the normal doses. It is effective in destroying the cancer cells, but it also destroys the bone marrow where essential blood cells are produced. To speed up the recovery of bone marrow and the production of healthy blood cells, Dr. Neidhart injects colony-stimulating factors (CSFs). I first heard of his work from several breast cancer patients who were pleased with their results.

Depending upon the treatment plan, patients need to remain in New Mexico for periods of a few weeks to several months. The center has arrangements with the motels in the area for moderate accommodations for patients and an accompanying family member or friend. Those patients who require longer stays can be put up at an apartment complex that offers special cancer center rates. The center will cover the housing costs depending upon the patient's need and ability to pay. Help with the local transportation and other needs are available through the center's Social Services Department. Other CCCs offering high intensity chemotherapy with CSFs can be located through the NCI PDQ system.

Dr. Isaac Djerassi (about whom you'll read more in upcoming chapters) also uses, when indicated, immuno-therapies in conjunction with his administration of high-dose chemotherapies.

GENE THERAPY: A LOOK AT THE FUTURE

Advances in molecular biology in the 1980s led to a new understanding of DNA that holds the genetic code on all forms of life. This in turn led to the Food and Drug Administration (FDA) giving approval in the fall of 1990 for the use of gene therapy as an experimental treatment approach for advanced melanoma, a deadly skin cancer. These tests are being conducted under the direction of Dr. Steven Rosenberg and his gene research team at the National Cancer Institute.

In the experimental procedure, a gene that tells the cell to produce TNF (tumor necrosis factor), a substance known to destroy tumors, is inserted into white blood cells taken from melanoma patients. In the following two weeks, the patient will be re-injected with billions of these geneti-cally altered cells which are expected to destroy or shrink the malignant growth.

LABORATORIES

Since cancer diagnosis, prognosis and management depends upon the expertise of the pathologists who interpret the initial laboratory tests, it is important to know that unique laboratories exist that do very sophisticated and exciting tests using the latest technology. They have flow cytometry, multidrug resistance testing, receptor analysis and many other tests and indexes that are not commonly available in many laboratories or small community hospitals. Their specialists have impressive credentials with extensive experience in interpreting the results of these highly technical tests.

One such laboratory is Dianon Systems, Inc., 200 Watson Boulevard, Stratford, Connecticut 06497. The telephone number is (203) 381-4000 or 1-800-328-2666. The company reports having a Cancer Management Program for breast, ovarian, and prostate cancers that can accurately diagnose, predict survival by distinguishing between high- and low-risk tumors, guide treatment, and monitor therapy by detecting early recurrence through a follow-up biomarker system.

Dianon's Prostate Cancer Management Program operates in conjunction with its partner laboratory Aspiration Biopsy Laboratory (ABL), which has performed over 50,000 readings on needle aspiration specimens and is the first national cancer reference laboratory. ABL performs DNA analysis for prostate cancer which provides vital information for the successful management of prostate cancer patients. Ask your physician about these tests, or you can call Dianon yourself and tell them your condition or what your physician suspects, to hear what the laboratory recommends in the way of tests.

Such laboratories are a viable way to go, especially if you are being treated for cancer at a small community hospital at a great distance from a medical center and in a very isolated area or at any general hospital whose pathology laboratory is not equipped with flow cytometry or other such technologies. I am sure any competent physician would welcome the value of the information from these sophisticated, predictive and case management tests.

Similar technology can be found at Cytometrics, Inc., 3520 Dunhill Street, San Diego, California 92121. The telephone number is 1-800-621-3321. Cytometrics, a division of Specialty Laboratories, Inc., provides comprehensive oncology testing services for physicians and hospitals and other reference laboratories. They report their professionals regularly attend conferences and educational programs and work closely with universities, private research laboratories and pharmaceutical companies to assist in research and development.

Another West Coast laboratory, with service centers across the country, is Nichols Institute, 33608 Ortega Highway, San Juan Capistrano, California 92690-6130. Nichols has been a source of the latest diagnostic and prognostic technologies to physicians and hospitals throughout the country. They also sponsor conferences and hands-on workshops to help educate physicians and technologists in utilizing new diagnostic and prognostic methods.

The value of having your analysis done at a laboratory such as Nichols Institute is that they have worked closely with the research community for years, and their list of Academic Associates is impressive. One example of their research collaboration is with Dr. William L. McGuire, Chief, Division of Medical Oncology, The University of Texas Health Sciences Center whose career has spanned 30 years of breast cancer research. The advantage of the medical testing is that during 20 years of operation they have interpreted large numbers of results. Since cancer testing can be very complicated and seldom involves black and white decisions, their access to large numbers of test results coupled with their extensive association with outstanding research, gives them the ability to tie in what those numbers mean and to sort out what they know about many patients and relate it to the result they get on a particular cancer test to come up with a more accurate interpretation. With this in mind, I urge you to *challenge* your doctors to investigate where is the best place for your tests. Don't accept pat answers.

With the explosion of technologies, you can expect laboratories such as these to be abreast of the latest developments and to be one of the first to offer them to the public.

. . . PERSONAL PERSPECTIVE

ह्ल

As I was into my final edit of the manuscript for this book, I was invited to join a group that was being formed to enlist volunteers to become bone marrow transplant donors. The group, the National Jewish Children's Leukemia Foundation, Inc., will conduct drives across the nation to enlist volunteers for the Bone Marrow Donors Program. This organization will fundraise to cover the cost of the initial blood testing of potential bone marrow donors.

The foundation was established by Tzvi Shor, whose son Meir was in desperate need of a bone marrow transplant. Since he couldn't find a match through family members, he was told that his next best chance to find a match was from someone of the same ethnic or racial background. Shor was also told that there is a severe shortage of donors from such minority groups as Jews, blacks, and Hispanics.

While searching for a match for his son, Mr. Shor raised the necessary funds to conduct seven drives in Jewish communities and enlisted close to 3,000 potential donors. He was fortunate; the intensive search produced a suitable match for Meir. In addition, a match for two other patients was found, and the names of close to 3,000 other volunteer donors were added to the National Marrow Donor Program Registry, which is mentioned in Chapter 9. The marrow will be available to patients of all faiths.

The purpose of establishing this program was so that Jews and other minority groups could be given a better chance of finding a suitable match.

There are more than 9,000 individuals who are in life-threatening danger and are desperately searching for a donor. For many, time is running out. Mr. Shor is anxious to get this message across to potential donors and to let them know that the process of donating bone marrow is quite uncomplicated. It starts with a simple blood test — and that could save a life.

The address of the foundation is 1310 48th Street, Brooklyn, New York 11219. The telephone number is (718) 853-0510.

Chapter 7

THE FINANCIAL QUEST:
THERE'S HELP

Many of the treatments I write about may be offered at a center far from your home. Because of family needs or other reasons, you may decide not to go to these centers. Others may want to go but can't afford it. What do you do if you can't afford it? Here are some options.

When you send your records to a cancer center or to a particular physician or consulting team for a second opinion, you may be told that only a slight variation is necessary and that your local oncologist can carry it out. On the other hand, if you are told, "We have some promising treatments for your type of malignancy, and we think we can help," I would certainly consider how to get to that facility quickly.

NEST EGG FOR
A RAINY DAY
ह➤

One of the most common responses I hear is, "I don't have the money. How can I afford all this costly treatment?" Maybe you have some money put away for a family vacation or your child's education. What about the little bit you've stashed away for retirement? Tell yourself that you're worth it and use the family nest egg. Ask yourself: What would I say about the use of the family's reserves if it were for a close family member instead of myself? Chances are your answer would be, "Go for it." Or think of what you would do if a member of your immediate family planned to get married in a faraway place? When they don't have choices, many people simply pack up and go without regard for expense.

CORPORATIONS WITH A HEART

For those who don't dare touch what they have set aside, or don't have any savings, there are people out there willing to help. The Corporate Angels Network (CAN) at (914) 328-1313 (see Appendix VI) provides transportation, when space is available, to cancer treatment centers on executive jet flights. CAREFORCE, based in Houston, Texas, a not-for-profit group of volunteers, most of whom have or have had an affiliation with Continental Airlines, fundraise within the community to help defer the costs of air travel for children and their families and other cancer patients when it is necessary for them to seek treatment some distance from their homes. Continental Airlines allots the organization 20 certificates a month which can be used toward a trip voucher. To initiate a request for help, call Continental Airlines toll-free number 1-800-525-0280 and ask for the current CAREFORCE telephone reference number. Malia Reed, president of this organization, reported that they have helped patients from as far away as Ecuador and Manila.

Ronald McDonald Houses, an international network (in nine countries) of accommodations located near many cancer centers, are available for family members to stay in while they have a seriously ill child receiving treatment at a nearby hospital. Families are asked to donate $5 to $15 per day. If it is not possible, the stay is free. Reservations can be made only through a referral from the hospital, so check with the social services department to see if there is a nearby facility.

HELP AT THE CENTERS

Many centers have special programs to help you meet medical costs. The Children's Caring Cancer Center at the University of Miami's Sylvester CCC provides financial assistance to many children. They will pay for medical treatment, including chemotherapy, radiation, laboratory work and clinic visits for any child who does not have insurance coverage. Even if a family has insurance, the Caring Cancer Center will help with the 20 percent difference. The Deed Club is committed to the support of the University of Miami's Bone Marrow Transplant Unit. St. Jude Children's Research Hospital in Memphis also offers financial aid to needy patients who meet grant requirements. The City of Hope near Los Angeles sometimes admits eligible patients to clinical trial programs free of charge. Most patients at cancer centers who are treated with costly experimental anti-cancer drugs receive them at no charge. Support like this does much to enhance the state of mind of patients and their families.

Insurance companies haven't paid for bone marrow transplantation in the past because it was considered experimental. However, bone marrow replacement is now state-of-the-art treatment for some of the blood cancers and for relapsed Hodgkin's disease and non-Hodgkin's lymphoma. Therefore, it is advisable that you check with your insurance company regarding eligible coverage. Some carriers are paying in part for bone marrow transplants in the treatment of breast cancer because it is often the treatment of choice when it has spread to other areas from the breast. Bone marrow transplant is being investigated as a treatment for many of the complicated or metastatic cancers, so the insurance picture may change.

If you need a bone marrow transplant and your insurance won't cover it, you may want to follow up on this lead. In September of 1991, I was told that the Children's Emergency Relief Foundation was being established to provide financial support for surgeries or procedures that are not covered by insurance. The Foundation will also provide medical equipment and home health aids to those who qualify. The address is: Post Office Box 28785, Atlanta, Georgia 30358; telephone: (404) 393-9474.

Meanwhile, if you have lost your hair from chemotherapy or radiation therapy and you need to purchase a wig or toupee, submit the invoice with the prescription and letter from your doctor to your insurance carrier. It should be covered.

Many insurance policies cover most of the costs of treating cancer. Some don't. But even if you have no insurance at all, you can work with your doctor, hospital or social worker to try to make financial arrangements that you can handle.

Check out the center where you want to get treatment. If it is in another state far from your home, some hospitals provide sleeping accommodations for a family member in the patient's room and the use of hospital kitchen facilities where he or she can prepare his/her own meals. This is a big saving. Eating out can further increase expenses. Other centers recommend moderately-priced sleeping accommodations nearby, and some centers have vans that provide transportation to and from the hospital. Ask your clergy to help locate a family in the area that could provide sleeping quarters or bed and board at nominal cost. Your church, temple, or synagogue may also have funds available for these purposes. Many service groups such as the Masons, Lions, Rotary, Kiwanis, the American Cancer Society, United Way, and other social agencies may be able to help.

HELP CLOSE
TO HOME
ફ✍

Patients who are eligible can apply for Medicare or Supplementary Security Insurance (SSI) or Medicaid and can check with the local Social Security office to see if their illness qualifies them for disability benefits, even if they are younger than 65.

In Florida, other benefits are available through Health Rehabilitative Services (HRS), which is the umbrella for a large variety of programs. Medicaid is administered through HRS as well as Aid for Dependent Children. When children qualify for the latter, they usually do for the former as well. Though there are limits on what they cover for adults, the caps for children (birth to age 21) has been lifted. It is difficult to give any dollar-and-cents figures as to the benefits since it varies from state to state. Under some Medicaid systems, you may be entitled to have home health attendants.

Another source of help is the Children's Medical Services (CMS), a state agency that gets partial support from the government. Children (newborn to age 21) with longterm chronic illnesses receive financial support from CMS. This includes patients with any type of cancer, if the family meets the criteria for federal poverty guidelines. Even for families that don't meet the poverty criteria, if the medical expenses are very high, I was told that the agency in Miami will do a financial review to determine the eligibility of the child. In any state, this agency can be located under your state listings in your telephone book.

If you have been hospitalized and are being released, speak with a hospital social worker to find out what benefits are available to you. The Visiting Nurse Service is available if you qualify. Check with your physician since he makes the decision and has to order the service. The Visiting Nurse Service in turn can order home health aids for a limited time.

I also checked with the Archdiocese of Miami and was told that though they have no ministry established to handle the express needs of cancer patients and their families, the Ministry on Grieving would certainly be a valid place to get some help as would be their Family Service Program. Several of the people I spoke with at the Archdiocese agreed that the place to start is the nearest church. One woman stressed that if patients or their families got a negative response from their local priest they needed to move on to one at another church. As she put it, "If you don't get results from one priest — *shop around until you do!*"

Ask your physician if you can expect to receive blood transfusions. If so, check with your family and friends regarding donating blood or find out what is the policy at the American Red Cross. This could amount to considerable savings. Inquire at your hospital's blood bank about preparing blood in advance or their replacement policies.

Most of the medical centers mentioned have clinics where the same physicians who treat private patients will see patients who cannot afford private care. A major problem a patient faces at some clinics is the life-threatening delays in diagnosis and treatment because the backlog is so great.

If this is the case and you are unable to see a physician or to have the necessary diagnostic tests within a month or so, keep going back. Be persistent. And if you have been diagnosed and need surgery or another type of treatment and it didn't get scheduled within four to six weeks, keep returning. Don't wait for an appointment. Tell them it's urgent. Tell them it's an emergency. Speak to a nurse supervisor. Enlist the help of a social worker. Persevere and keep showing up until you do get the attention and care that you need.

On the positive side, most clinics provide excellent care and patients are seen within a reasonable amount of time. When I was treated at Dana-Farber in Boston, I spoke with several patients who were unable to pay for the services who nevertheless were treated with the same dignity and excellent medical treatment as paying patients. As you read in Chapter 5, Columbia-Presbyterian CCC Ambulatory Oncology Center in New York City provides cancer care to all patients in need. Look for centers such as these. They are around.

Medical care is expensive. Worry over astronomical bills from hospitals and specialists is additional stress the patient doesn't need. Don't let yourself get tied up in knots over money. Go for the best treatment available, and then

work out the details of paying for it. You may not be aware
of all the available options.

... PERSONAL PERSPECTIVE

ह~

*Our insurance covered most of my medical expenses,
but we had no idea of how high our expenses might go —
because of our uncertainties, we didn't spend too freely on
the household needs. I surely could have used more help
with the macrobiotic cooking. It was very difficult, very
time-consuming, and physically draining. I should have let
friends, many of whom offered, lighten my burden, but
Seymore and I had always been responsible for ourselves,
and I didn't know what it was like to let people help.*

*I was like many people who were used to taking care of
their own needs. They don't know how to ask for help; they
don't know how to accept help. Most don't even want it
known that they could use help. I had to learn how to take
from others. And I'm grateful to all my friends who made it
so easy for me.*

*I was especially grateful to my husband Seymore
because he never objected to all the plane fares to Boston for
my tests and treatments. There were times when he might
complain about an expensive flight to attend a wedding or
other function, but he never questioned my spending when
it was for health purposes. Getting the best medical care was
a top priority for both of us. Today I feel sure that this was
a strong factor in my recovery.*

Chapter 8

TANGLING WITH TOUGH TUMORS:
HELP FOR HARD-TO-TREAT CANCERS

If the idea of a hospital devoted to cancer care conjures up visions of suffering and depression, you haven't visited a Comprehensive Cancer Center. In these enclaves where cancer is a fact of life, the general feeling is optimistic. Armed with a cheerful attitude and formidable knowledge, staff members daily meet the enemy without fear. They are accustomed to miracles. With all their expertise in so many areas of treating cancer, they are especially concerned about the patient's welfare.

There are more than 100 different kinds of cancer. There are rare or hard-to-treat varieties as well as those that respond well to state-of-the-art approaches.

For those with a rare or complicated cancer, CCCs offer another important, if intangible, element: *reason to hope.* Even if you never considered this before, even if you've been through other treatments that were not effective, it is never too late. Perhaps there is help for you on the cutting edge.

Yet it is important to know that there are other factors (such as the stage or advancement of the cancer and if there has been metastasis and to what extent it is) involved in what determines whether a normally easy-to-treat cancer would require the expertise of a research-oriented cancer center.

A brief overview of many centers' advances in the treatment of a few of the more common cancers that are hard to treat will show you how hope comes from knowledge. Remember that methods available at one Comprehensive Cancer Center may be offered at all or most of the others. Yet, bear in mind also that in some instances a more highly qualified specialist or a unique treatment may be found at a center known for its expertise in treating a particular type of cancer.

Here's a sampling of the possibilities:

BLADDER CANCER:

ટ♥

Doctors are now able to install an internal collection device in patients whose cancer necessitates removal of the bladder. The first artificial bladder was the Koch pouch. This device and other modifications provide patients with alternatives to an external collection bag. The right colon pouch, which reduced surgery time and patient discomfort, was developed in 1987. A year later, a team of specialists at Columbia-Presbyterian Medical Center developed a major modification that resulted in further reduction of surgery time and risk of incontinence. The initial two pouches used some of the lower small intestine to create an artificial bladder, but the Columbia innovation was a bladder fashioned from the colon only. This eliminates the risk of malabsorption of nutrients [since the lower small intestine plays an important role in digestion]. The Columbia team has added additional modifications, but still further refinement is necessary. If you are a candidate for bladder surgery, you should discuss with your doctor the procedure *before* the surgery takes place.

BONE CANCER:

ટ♥

Osteosarcoma, a bone cancer that strikes adolescents, is responding well in trials at a number of cancer centers. A 15-year study at Dana-Farber and Memorial Sloan-Kettering showed that chemotherapy used after surgery boosts the survival rate from 20 percent to 60-80 percent in those bone cancers that have not spread. Other centers reporting a high success rate in this type of cancer include Roswell Park (Buffalo, New York), the University of Miami (Florida), and Yale.

Limb-preservation techniques — such as a tourniquet infusion method of high-dose chemotherapy used at Roswell Park and other centers — enable bone cancer patients, for whom amputation was once inevitable, to lead normal lives. This is a procedure whereby high-dose chemotherapy is delivered to the limb below the tourniquet while the blood flow to the rest of the body is blocked. This limits the topic effects of high-dose chemotherapy to the body and is thus able to preserve the limb. Memorial Sloan-Kettering reports that combined therapies are used to cure patients with soft-tissue cancer of an arm or leg and at the same time to preserve the affected limb. The therapies include surgery to remove the tumor, radiation and chemotherapy to prevent local recurrence of the tumor, and chemotherapy to destroy cancer cells that may have spread beyond the original site.

At the University of Miami, which boasts one of the country's largest tissue banks, doctors use biologic substitutes for bones and joints to replace tumorous bones. This is a big improvement over metal replacements. Dr. B. E. Buck with the Tissue Bank of the Department of Orthopedics and Rehabilitation, University of Miami, explained that when they preserve bone for a transplant, they deliberately kill the bone cells by freezing the bone and attempt to wash out all the bone marrow and fat. Because of the freezing, there is no problem with rejection. If they were to transplant fresh bone, it is rejected. In this type of bone transplant, the recipient's living bone grows into and slowly fuses with the bone graft. The transplanted bone is not going to break up. The only thing we tell our patients, said Dr. Buck, is, "Don't run, that's all."

In the early 70s, Dr. Isaac Djerassi together with Dr. Norman Jaffe — who was then at Children's Hospital in Boston and is now at M. D. Anderson in Houston — perfected the application of high-dose methotrexate, an anti-cancer agent, to raise the survival rate of patients with osteogenic sarcoma — a deadly bone cancer — from 20 percent to 60 percent. Dr. Isaac Djerassi, a pioneer in the use of high-dose methotrexate, is the director of the Cancer Mini-Center at Mercy Catholic Medical Center Misericordia Hospital at 54th and Cedar Avenue, Philadelphia, Pennsylvania 19143. Dr. Djerassi's telephone number is (215) 748-9180.

BRAIN CANCER:

Research in brain cancer treatment is equally dramatic and diverse.

Columbia-Presbyterian Medical Center in New York City, which has a well-deserved reputation for exceptional expertise in treating many forms of cancer, is among the largest centers in research and treatment of brain tumors. Columbia is a center that reports the use of bone marrow transplantation to treat certain types of brain tumors as well as stereotactic radiation therapy.

The University of Wisconsin, noted for excellent work in treating childhood cancers, reported treating brain tumors in children and adults as well with stereotactic radiation. As you read in Chapter 6, this is a procedure whereby the surgeon attaches a frame to the head to permit precise positioning when necessary to allow for high doses of radiation to be delivered to the site of the tumor.

In 1985, Dr. Isaac Djerassi reported a high success rate using methotrexate for astrocytoma, the most common brain tumor. Dr. Vincent T. DeVita, Jr., then director of the National Cancer Institute (NCI), was quoted in the April 22, 1985, issue of *Medical World News* as saying, "I've never seen as many long-term survivors (percentage wise) as Dr. Djerassi is reporting." Previously, this form of cancer was found to be unresponsive to chemotherapy, but methotrexate crosses the blood-brain barrier (a system that limits which substances can enter the brain), while most drugs do not.

Dr. DeVita warns that "very high-dose methotrexate is not something the average doctor should embark on unless he's had a lot of experience." Thus, any patient needing high-dose methotrexate might be wise to go to a cancer center with this kind of expertise.

BREAST CANCER:
ॐ

The search for the best breast cancer treatment sparked one of the most intense medical controversies of the last few decades. In the 1950s, the introduction of the *lumpectomy* (removal of only the diseased portion of the breast and any affected lymph nodes as opposed to a mastectomy, traditional radical surgery involving removal of the entire breast), divided the medical community, though the lumpectomy was limited to selected patients with early stage breast cancer. Since then, both types of surgery, in combination with radiation and/or chemotherapy, have been state-of-the-art treatments.

In 1988, Dr. William Hrushesky when at the University of Minnesota discovered from his laboratory results of studies of mice with breast cancer that there might be a relationship between cancer survival and the time of initial surgery, with respect to the time of a woman's menstrual cycle. A later study reported in *Lancet*, October 21, 1989, by Dr. Hrushesky, who is now at the Stratton V.A. Medical Center in Albany, New York, confirmed his initial results. Further studies in this area have discovered that in women operated on for breast cancer as close as possible to the time of ovulation and during the week following it, the outcome was more successful in terms of survival time and the prevention of metastasis (spread of the disease).

Apparently, there is some connection between the hormones that are particularly active near and shortly after ovulation and the balance between a woman and her cancer. Since the menstrual cycle may be important to the scheduling of breast cancer surgery, women who are normally lax about keeping a calendar might benefit from keeping track. Further research could prove that an overall picture of a woman's menstrual cycle over the years might have significance.

Researchers at the University of Wisconsin pioneered (in this country) treating breast cancer patients with tamoxifen, an anti-estrogen drug. This hormonal therapy has exhibited no serious side effects and is now used in hospitals around the world.

Findings from three American studies testing tamoxifen on women with early breast cancer with negative nodes (meaning that the breast cancer has not spread to the lymph nodes) showed significant improvement in the rates of disease-free survival. These findings were consistent with long-term European studies.

Advances such as these prompted Dr. DeVita, who was then director of NCI, to make a definitive statement on May 18, 1988. He said that the state-of-the-art treatment for early stage breast cancer with no lymph node involvement is chemotherapy and/or hormonal therapy following the primary treatment by lumpectomy and radiation.

Women with breast cancer that has not spread to the lymph nodes could benefit from this treatment if they learned about it in time. This therapy needs to be given within a specific period after primary surgery or radiation. This is a prime example of the advantages of being part of a clinical trial. Women who were in the NCI trials received the more beneficial therapy long before it was made available to the general population. At the time of the announcement, scores of frightened, angry women jammed the telephone lines to question why they weren't given benefit of this successful treatment.

But this approach is not necessarily the way to go for every node negative breast cancer patient. As was mentioned, treatment protocols change from time to time. But one call to the CIS at 1-800-4-CANCER will keep you abreast of what is current. You can also ask about the outcome of projected clinical trials by the NCI in the use of taxol, a substance taken from the bark of the western yew tree, for advanced breast cancers.

CHILDHOOD LEUKEMIA:

The first remissions in this illness were achieved with the then-new technique of chemotherapy in the late 1940s by Dana-Farber founder Dr. Sidney Farber, who is often called the father of modern chemotherapy. To this day, the Dana-Farber Cancer Institute is at the forefront in treating childhood leukemia. The institute notes particular success with acute lymphocytic leukemia (ALL), a once-fatal form of the disease for which Dana-Farber records a 77-percent survival rate.

Researchers at St. Jude Children's Research Hospital in Memphis, the largest childhood cancer center in the world, have obtained good results treating acute lymphocytic leukemia patients with high-dose methotrexate. It is added to their conventional chemotherapy, which is followed by a *rescue* technique that protects healthy organs from harmful side effects.

Bone marrow transplantation is also widely used in the treatment of leukemia.

COLORECTAL CANCER:

Advances in diagnostic capabilities are making early detection of colon cancer easier. This allows patients to take advantage of advances in surgery. Techniques developed at Yale have reduced the need for colostomies (an opening outside of the body with a bag attached to collect bowel waste) by 80 percent for patients whose lower rectal cancer was diagnosed in the early stages. Mayo surgeons have refined ways of preserving normal function in patients who have rectal cancer surgery, thus greatly enhancing the lives of patients who might otherwise have needed to wear an external bag for the rest of their lives.

Most cancer center hospitals offer lower rectal surgeries that restore some function for patients in whom such operations are technically feasible. One expert advises that uncomplicated colon cancers can be removed surgically by any competent proctologist. When looking for answers for a hard-to-treat colon cancer, it might be helpful to check with the National Surgical Adjuvant Project for Breast and Bowel Cancers (NSABP), listed in Appendix III.

A breakthrough in rectal cancer was announced in March, 1991, by Dr. Samuel Broder, Director of the NCI. It was found that the use of the chemotherapy drug 5FU alone or in conjunction with other chemotherapies after surgery and radiation (standard treatment) reduced the death rate of rectal cancer to 38 percent — down from 59 percent in patients who received the surgery and radiation alone. One physician's comment on Dr. Broder's announcement was that there will still be some doctors who will say, "I know surgery alone is okay." — *Be careful you don't settle for a doctor who still thinks that way.*

LUNG CANCER:

Primary lung cancer is the major cause of cancer-related adult deaths in the United States. Yet, in the past 20 years, the approximate 10-12 percent five-year survival rate has not changed.

Extensive drug sensitivity studies are being conducted at the NCI's laboratories to test the effectiveness of selected chemotherapies against non-small-cell lung cancer. This accounts for 75 percent of lung cancers and is relatively resistant to chemotherapy. Small-cell, or oat-cell lung cancer is a very fast-growing type, although major advances have been made in the treatment of the disease using chemotherapy and radiotherapy. One of the biggest mistakes a physician can make is to assume that when a lung cancer spreads, nothing more can be done. This robs the patient of all hope and sends the message that the only option is to die with dignity. In fact, cooperative oncology teams avail themselves of current research and are every patient's best source of hope.

Dr. Edward J. Beattie, a skilled thoracic surgeon at Beth Israel Hospital in New York City, reports that lung cancer is a very complicated cancer that needs to be treated by a highly qualified team comprised of an oncological surgeon, a radiation oncologist and a medical oncologist working as partners rather than in isolation. There are fourteen different stages or types of lung cancer so the team needs to know what it is doing. As part of a research project, Dr. Beattie orders chemosensitivity assay testing of malignant tissue at the time of surgery for patients who have advanced cancer and are apt to need chemotherapy.

He has worked together with Dr. Djerassi, a medical oncologist in Philadelphia, who first treats a patient with chemotherapy to shrink the tumor. If the tumor is not removable, Dr. Beattie then performs lung surgery in conjunction with internal radiation therapy which is delivered directly into the site of the tumor at the time of surgery by the radiation team. This team is headed by Dr. Bhadrasain Vikram, Chief of the Radiation Department, a skilled and experienced radiation therapist who was the designated head and neck specialist in the Department of Radiation Oncology at Memorial-Sloan Kettering for twelve years.

Lung cancer is still a disaster. There are 158,000 new cases a year with 143,000 deaths. This is a cure rate of ten percent. Of course, smoking accounts for 80 percent of those cases. The other side of the coin, Dr. Beattie pointed out, is those lung cancers that are under three centimeters when diagnosed can boast an 85-percent cure rate, assuming there has been no spread. Forty percent of such tumors can be detected with an annual chest X-ray. With hopeful statistics like these, heavy smokers might want to ask themselves, "When did I have my last chest X-ray?"

MELANOMA:

ﱞﺝ

Still one of the most difficult cancers to treat, melanoma is the subject of numerous clinical trials around the country, some with promising results. The Yale Cancer Center is one of the top melanoma units in the country, and the University of Pennsylvania's Pigmented Lesion Clinic (which treats more than 2,500 melanoma patients a year), is recognized as one of the world's premier melanoma clinics.

After more than 20 years of multidisciplinary research, experts at the Kaplan Cancer Center at New York University have been able to identify those malignant melanoma patients who are at high risk for having their cancer spread. This is important. When surgeons remove the primary tumor identified in the disease's early stages, malignant melanoma is often cured.

But when melanoma recurs and spreads beyond the skin, it usually becomes particularly virulent and hard to treat. Dr. Jean-Claude Bystryn of NYU constructed his own melanoma vaccine which is still in clinical trials. It may prevent recurrence of malignant melanoma in high-risk patients. The vaccine is based on an immunotherapeutic agent that doctors think might inhibit or arrest secondary tumor nodules, lumps or knots of cells once they appear. Dr. Bystryn uses immune markers to measure the vaccine's ability to stimulate an immune response to melanoma.

Other melanoma vaccines have been developed and extensive testing of these vaccines is being conducted at many other centers so there is a good possibility of finding one near your home if you wish to look into this type of treatment.

In Chapter 6, you read of hyperthermia, the use of high heat to treat tumors, in combination with anti-cancer agents and with radiation. Several cancer centers report that it is being investigated as a treatment modality for melanoma.

It was reported in Chapter 5 that IL-2 was an effective treatment for certain advanced melanoma patients. And you read in Chapter 6 about Dr. Steven Rosenberg, of the NCI, who conducted the first trials in May, 1991, using gene therapy to treat advanced malignant melanoma. This is used in combination with immunotherapy and is expected to enhance the outcome of treatment.

And in November, 1991, the Albert Einstein Cancer Center in the Bronx reported clinical trials conducted by Dr. Avi Einzig, Associate Professor of Medicine, and Dr. Peter H. Wiernik, Associate Director of the Center, with taxol, a substance taken from the bark of a western yew tree. The taxol studies have been conducted with melanoma and ovarian cancers and have had promising results.

Further trials in melanoma, ovarian, breast and other cancers are in progress at other centers also in this new and exciting drug.

It is still too soon to know the usefulness of these trials, but the Cancer Information Service (CIS) toll-free number *1-800-4-CANCER* is a good place to call to keep abreast of what is happening with the trials or to locate a center that offers one or more of these treatments.

The American Cancer Society recommends a monthly inspection of your skin. Any mole with irregular edges can be an early melanoma, which in this early stage is highly curable. Since melanoma is difficult to put into remission once it spreads, potential candidates for treatment should be eager to look into various aspects of research.

Those interested in updates or more extensive information on melanoma or skin cancer can contact the Skin Cancer Foundation, 245 Fifth Avenue, Suite 2402, New York, NY 10016, (212) 725-5176. They have several publications available for patient and public education. They also publish the *Melanoma Letter,* a superb newsletter directed more specifically to the melanoma patient.

OVARIAN CANCER:
   ࿓

Still very difficult to treat, ovarian cancer is the subject of multicenter studies that are investigating various treatment methods. One of the big problems with this type of cancer is that by the time it is diagnosed it is usually in an advanced stage and is hard to treat. The Columbia-Presbyterian Medical Center in New York City reports studies that use transvaginal sonography to evaluate menopausal women at risk for ovarian cancer. The researchers believe that this test, together with the CA-125 blood test, may be effective in identifying early ovarian cancers.

An important source of information is the Familial Ovarian Cancer Registry established in 1981 by M. Steven Piver, M.D., Chief of the Department of Gynecologic Oncology at Roswell Park Cancer Institute, Elm and Carlton Streets, Buffalo, NY 14263, telephone: 1-800-OVARIAN. In

May, 1990, actor Gene Wilder, was made honorary chairman of the Registry. It was renamed the Gilda Radner Familial Ovarian Cancer Registry in honor of his comedienne wife who died of ovarian cancer in 1989. Mr. Wilder firmly believes that had his wife known of the family link in ovarian cancer and had access to Dr. Piver and his knowledge of the disease, she would be alive today.

The problem with detecting the disease in its early stage is that the symptoms can be vague. The most common complaints of feeling tired, bloated or having abdominal pain and backaches are confusing because women who don't have ovarian cancer often feel that way, too. The important thing is to see your doctor if the symptoms persist or if they get worse. Pelvic examination, pelvic ultrasound and the CA-125 blood test identify the possibility of ovarian cancer. Though these tests are not foolproof, they need to be used together to be effective. Bear in mind that the disease is comparatively rare and survival rates are very good for those ovarian cancers that are detected early.

Intraperitoneal (intra-abdominal) administration of anti-cancer agents (see Chapter 5), as well as the use of immune boosters like interleukin-2, are treatments being used at present. But the facts are not all in and the treatments for ovarian cancer are by no means conclusive. As you've read in Chapter 5, promising results have been shown in clinical trials using taxol, obtained from the bark of a western yew tree, to test ovarian cancer. Because of the frequent changes expected in the multicenter studies, it is wise to put in a *query* through PDQ at the CIS.

Laparotomy, second-look surgery, is often performed after standard therapy to determine if any of the original tumor has remained. If you've been treated for ovarian cancer, you might want to ask your oncologist if you are a candidate for laparotomy. If so, be sure of the experience factor of the surgeon who will perform the procedure.

OTHER CANCERS

The list goes on. Dr. Alfred S. Ketcham, Chief of Surgical Oncology at the University of Miami, is co-developer of an operation named for him. The Ketcham Procedure combines the expertise of a neurosurgeon and a head and neck surgeon, both working to eradicate tumors of the facial and skull sinuses that have invaded the brain.

Pancreatic cancers have been treated surgically, with immune boosters, with bone marrow transplants, and with intraoperative radiation and hyperthermia.

Laser therapy has proved palliative (effective for reducing pain) for *cancer of the esophagus* at the Ireland Center, and at Fox Chase, esophageal cancer has been treated with a combination of chemotherapy and radiation without sacrificing the esophagus. The patients remained disease-free for more than three years.

Dr. Muhyi Al-Sarraf, Director of Head, Neck and Esophagus Departments at Wayne State University Comprehensive Cancer Center in Detroit pointed out in a telephone interview that researchers at Fox Chase CCC, the University of Rochester Clinical Cancer Center, and Wayne State University were involved in the initial trials that established combination chemotherapy and radiation as state-of-the-art treatment for esophageal cancer. Dr. Al-Sarraf reported it can take as long as ten years for the results of a clinical trial to get to the community level. This is the advantage of being treated at a comprehensive or clinical cancer center. You are in on the ground floor.

Dr. Edward J. Beattie, of Beth-Israel Hospital in New York City, reports the 17-year survival of a patient with cancer of the esophagus.

Surgery alone, radiation implants, surgery combined with drugs and radiation, the combination of chemotherapy and radiation and hyperthermia and radiation or chemotherapy all hold promise for treating *head and neck cancers*.

To write about the hundreds of on-going clinical trials being investigated at this time on the hard-to-treat and complicated cancers would be counter-productive. Instead,

I have limited this discussion to a few centers that have reported doing research or conducting trials on several of the hard-to-treat cancers. You may want simply to look at a center that is geographically convenient. If they are no longer involved in that area of research or treatment, it is more than likely that they are investigating another pro-tocol (method of treatment) for the same type of cancer. When a cancer center has invested a great deal of time and money to study a particular form of the disease and that research has not paid off, the center will generally go on to develop further studies of the same cancer.

All this is not meant to negate the outstanding specialists found at dozens of other institutions. In Boston alone, besides the NCI-approved Dana-Farber Cancer Institute, you will find some of the most qualified physicians in the world at hospitals like Massachusetts General, New England Deaconess, Beth Israel, Brigham and Women's, The University Hospitals, and more. New York, Chicago, Los Angeles, San Francisco, Kansas City, St. Louis, Texas, and other areas noted for their medical centers have their own highly qualified specialists. Not to be overlooked are the many outstanding oncologists who have been trained at top medical facilities and can be found in private practice throughout the country.

You already know that the NCI awards grants to cancer researchers and cancer centers, oversees the quality of research and treatment, and sets the standards that designated cancer centers must maintain. But the Division of Cancer Treatment of the NCI also conducts hundreds of clinical trials in its own facilities in Bethesda and Frederick, Maryland. This division develops new treatment approaches and evaluates new cancers.

These descriptions of cancer research are just a few examples of the diversity of possible options. You can't begin to select a treatment based on this information alone, because it is, of necessity, brief, but it gives you an idea of what is out there. Meanwhile, there are hundreds of reasons to ask your doctor to find out what is being tested at cancer centers. A new treatment might affect you.

Cancer research is moving forward constantly. Clinical trials will show that some treatments don't work; others will prove that new approaches are effective. Since my research began, at least two major breakthroughs have occurred. One resulted in hormonal therapy or chemotherapy being added to the standard lumpectomy and radiation protocol for early-diagnosed breast cancer. The second called for the use of chemotherapy with 5FU after surgery and radiation for rectal cancers. This is what every cancer patient waits for — the big breakthrough that will put his or her cancer into remission, that will improve the odds of surviving.

. . . PERSONAL PERSPECTIVE

I think my acceptance into Dana-Farber Cancer Institute's clinical trial of high-dose methotrexate, in combination with aggressive chemotherapy, was a turning point in my life. At that time my type of lymphoma was still considered hard-to-treat.

Dr. Emil Frei, III, explained to me that my condition was serious. My lymphoma was in an advanced (third) stage. With great enthusiasm, he explained that 70 percent of patients who followed the protocol he was recommending to me survived for a year and a half. Fifty percent of that number, he said, made it through the crucial first five years. He looked at me with a big smile and said, "Isn't that great?"

I forced a weak smile. Inside my head, I was screaming: "What are you talking about, Doctor? I was just 48 when this thing started. My sons are only teenagers!"

In the midst of my initial shock and fright, I tried to compose myself and ask Dr. Frei some sensible questions. "What happened to that half of the 70 percent after they made it to the five-year mark?"

He told me that the treatment plan was still experimental; there weren't any data available beyond five years. His confidence and enthusiasm were so infectious that, although I was shaken to the core, I blurted, "With the help of God, Doctor, I'll write pages in your medical records every year 'til I'm 120!"

Chapter 9

BECOMING AN EXPERT:

HOW TO RESEARCH YOUR OWN CASE

These are exciting times in cancer research, a battle that attracts some of the best minds in modern medicine. Cancers considered incurable today may be controlled tomorrow.

After any cancer diagnosis, you need state-of-the-art treatment. After diagnosis of a complicated, rare or hard-to-treat cancer, you may need to bring your case to the leading edge of cancer research. Investigating your own case is one way you can be sure of getting the best, most specific care.

Before we discuss new drugs, finding a qualified specialist and some other special resources, there are critical steps you may want to take before having a biopsy, such as those you read about in Chapter 6, and you know they must be addressed *before* the biopsy.

If your physician orders a biopsy of a tumor to determine if it is malignant or because there is a suspicion that a cancer has recurred or spread, this is a time to discuss who will interpret the pathology studies. This is done by a pathologist, to put it simply, a medical doctor trained to study body tissue to make a diagnosis or to predict the expected outcome of the disease. It is also time to ask if it is appropriate to get a second interpretation at a qualified laboratory that can do more extensive tests and whose pathologists have more experience and expertise. Similarly, if a diagnosis of cancer is made but the pathologist cannot identify the site of origin, this is the time for technology such as flow cytometry to do the specialized analyses you read about in Chapter 6. Remember that the site of origin is crucial to selection of the best treatment plan.

I know of several cases of a new cancer that were treated with drugs appropriate for the original cancer. The assumption was that the second cancer was a metastasis (a result of the spread) of the first tumor. In one instance, laboratory studies later revealed that the second cancer was entirely new and might have responded to a totally different group of anti-cancer drugs than those that were used. After the faulty diagnosis was realized and the patient was given the correct treatment, it was too late.

FINDING THE LATEST TREATMENTS

ટ≫

It was reported by *The Miami News* on June 30, 1987, that Dr. Bruce A. Chabner of the National Cancer Institute (NCI) told the Home Energy and Commerce Health Subcommittee that the best care is not made available to many cancer patients because their doctors are not up-to-date on the latest research developments. The NCI regularly mails new treatment information to doctors, but "whether the physicians read it and take it to heart is another matter," says Dr. Chabner.

Many doctors are unwilling to use NCI's information resources because using the newest treatment plans might involve them in the bureaucratic logistics of a clinical trial. Until the Food and Drug Administration (FDA) officially approves a new drug, any physician who uses it is considered part of the research team and must write detailed reports on every step of the patient's progress, or lack of it. Because of this extra record-keeping, paperwork and redtape, many doctors stay with the established treatment plan. But routine treatment may not always be enough for the rare or hard-to-treat cancers.

The process of researching your cancer is somewhat complicated. To find the best treatment, you can begin with a telephone call to NCI's computerized reference service called Physician's Data Query (PDQ), discussed in Chapter 4.

Unfortunately, many doctors who treat cancer are not diligent about using PDQ. Perhaps it just hasn't become a working habit. I've met many doctors who treat cancer patients and don't know that PDQ exists. I mentioned it to one of them who kept insisting that I meant the *PDR, Physicians' Desk Reference,* a standard book on medications. But when I discussed it with another doctor, he queried the service about a particularly stubborn cancer case he was treating. The service gave him some promising leads, and he couldn't thank me enough for the information. Most doctors are responsive once they become aware of this valuable source.

Originally, only doctors could call PDQ. But recognizing the urgent need to share information about cancer, former NCI director Dr. Vincent T. DeVita, Jr., opened PDQ to the public — a welcome innovation.

When you call the NCI's Cancer Information Service (CIS) toll-free number, 1-800-4-CANCER, to request a PDQ search on a particular cancer, you receive a run-down of the most up-to-date information available. Before a PDQ search can be conducted, there are several points of information about the specific case that must be provided: the type of cancer, the stage to which it has developed, and the forms of treatment, if any, that have been employed. Most patients know these details of their own case, but if the information is needed, it can be obtained from your physician's records.

You'll get a lot of information, only some of which is relevant to your case, but dig through until you find what you need. Whether you have a treatable cancer or you need that one-in-a-million cure, leave no stone unturned.

Remember, though, that it's not fair to your doctors to rush to them with everything you've read or heard. To maintain the team approach, you may want to discuss with your oncologist some investigational trials or second opinions that you'd like to look into on your own. Then, armed with more complete information, you can get back to him to discuss what you have found. With his help, you can knowledgeably determine if any of these treatments might be relevant in your case. If not, what does the doctor suggest? Then research that area.

You will then want your oncologist to help you determine the most promising treatment plan for you. Invite him to do this, but bear in mind he has to charge appropriately for the time it takes. If you cannot afford a private physician and are being treated at a medical center clinic, you will probably be treated by a very qualified physician. But there is still no reason why you can't do some investigating on your own and discuss it with your clinic physician.

Of course, you don't have to follow any doctor's treatment suggestion. You always have a choice: comply, don't comply, or do nothing at all. But you must have confidence in your decision. Having the facts makes you confident.

Let's take a hypothetical case of an already diagnosed advanced melanoma and pursue a decision-making path.

* * * * *

1. Call CIS (1-800-4-CANCER) to find out what the cutting edge of treatment is for advanced melanoma. You will learn about studies on combating this, the most serious form of skin cancer, with interleukin-2 (IL-2) and lymphokine-activating killer (LAK) cells (see Chapters 5 and 8).

As you read in Chapter 5, studies of this form of treatment were conducted at NCI research facilities in 1988. Their outcome was twofold. First, they determined that IL-2 — with or without LAK cells — was, at that time, the most effective treatment for both advanced kidney cancer and certain types of advanced melanoma. These studies also led the NCI to approve six cancer centers to conduct additional research. That research, in turn, led to funding for a modified Group C clinical test program at designated cancer centers.

2. That's where you come in. Consider the list of

centers handling this clinical trial. Hold your breath — it's a long list, but that makes our decision-making drill more realistic. More than 23 comprehensive and clinical centers were designated to do this testing.

Remember, this is an exercise designed to give you an idea of how to go about doing this kind of research for yourself. When you look into your own case, you can refine your decision about which treatment you might pursue and which center you might visit. They are all outstanding.

The centers conducting these trials range in geographic diversity from Washington State to Vermont, from Detroit to Birmingham, Salt Lake City to Chapel Hill.

3. Once you've learned that relevant clinical trial programs exist, here are some points you may want to consider in your decision-making.

You can ask how many patients were treated, and for how long were they followed. Ask what percentage of patients had, for instance, a reduction in tumor size, how many went into remission, how many died, how many had their cancer spread, and how many dropped out because they could not tolerate the treatment?

4. The answers to these questions will give you a pretty good picture of how the patients are doing in this program. Then discuss the pros and cons with your family, your doctors, your counselor and other people you rely upon. Now you are ready to move toward making an informed decision, a confident choice. You are doing your job, fighting on your own behalf.

5. When you discuss this information with your oncologist, and if he suggests you enter one of these investigational trials, how do you decide which center to go to for treatment?

It is important to realize that in some cases, there will be only one center with an available opening in a test group, or you may not meet the criteria for that trial, but generally you'll be able to be at least slightly selective. The simplest alternative may be the center closest to your home, or the one with the most affordable program. If you need a family member with you, select a facility with on-site or nearby family quarters.

I included this example of the extensiveness of an NCI-sponsored investigational study for two reasons: to illustrate the decision-making process and to give an idea of how an improvement on standard treatment of a particular type of cancer can be found. It doesn't always happen that an improvement will be found, but in research this is the way breakthroughs come about.

As you read in Chapters 6 and 8, researchers may be on to another breakthrough in melanoma. Gene therapy is showing promise in the treatment of this disease but is still a long way from being available to the general public. It will first have to undergo rigorous trials as was done with the IL-2 studies discussed above. The same is true of taxol that we read about earlier.

There are a few more resources you can explore. PDQ will lead you to the National Cancer Institute's Clinical Trials Cooperative Group Program (CTCGP) — see Appendix III — which was mentioned in Chapter 8. Members of these participating groups work together to design carefully controlled investigational trials that utilize sophisticated techniques. Such trials are developed to test new anti-cancer agents that come out of the drug development program at the NCI and are conducted in a multi-institutional setting.

You might want to ask your oncologist to investigate a specific anti-cancer agent that is being tested. Your doctor may find that it is in too early a stage of development to be a realistic way for you to go. If it does appear to be appropriate, it may help to get a picture of what you might expect if you enter a particular trial. In some investigational trials, treatments have to be conducted with the patient in intensive care, side effects can be very serious and at times debilitating, but most appear to be reversible. Reading about these trials can be both frightening and encouraging. Patients may improve, survive longer or even experience a remission. And that is what every patient entering a clinical trial hopes for.

It's important to know what the potential side effects

are or can be. When you have been made aware of how you may feel after the treatment, then you can tell yourself, "I really feel like I'm not going to make it, but my doctor told me that I could expect this." With that knowledge, you can think positively and focus on the hope that this treatment offers. Most of the patients I counsel handle all the side effects well when they know what to expect.

Another resource, already described in Chapter 6, is the American Cancer Society (ACS), which sponsors many research projects and clinical trial programs. The nurse-educator at your local branch will have information about current trials for your type of cancer.

Philanthropic foundations, private health care institutions and well-to-do individuals or families often fund cancer research and trials. Much of this research is also supported by pharmaceutical companies. Your local cancer information service should be able to help you locate any relevant programs in your area.

Further, the NCI funds nine institutions to conduct initial studies of new drugs in their drug development program. If you have a rare cancer — one for which there are no established standard treatment protocols — you may find some answers in the realm of new drug testing.

The Mayo Clinic's Comprehensive Cancer Center is one of these nine new drug testing facilities. You or your oncologist can call to see if any of the drugs they are testing for NCI show promising results for your type of cancer.

FINDING A BONE
MARROW DONOR

In the case of *allogeneic bone marrow transplants*, finding a compatible bone marrow match has often meant an agonizing period of stress for the patient and the family. Thanks to funding through a contract with the National Heart, Lung and Blood Institute, the American Red Cross, the American Association of Blood Banks, and the Council of Community Blood Centers, the *National Marrow Donor Program* (NMDP) has been created to improve the donor search process. The address is 100 South Robert Street, St. Paul, Minnesota 55107. The telephone number is 1-800-654-1247 or (612) 627-5800. There is no charge for a preliminary search listing all potential matches on file. The fee will vary for a formal search, which would be more exact and involve more extensive laboratory testing. They report three to four months as being the average time to provide the donor marrow. It was suggested the physician or patient check the progress of the search with the transplant center.

To initiate a bone marrow search, the patient or physician would have to call a transplant center. There are 29 National Marrow Donor Program Transplant Centers affiliated with the NMDP. Names and addresses can be requested from the National Marrow Donor Program at the telephone number listed above.

You can contact other registries through American Association of Bone Marrow Donor Registries, c/o The Caitlin Raymond International Registry of Bone Marrow Donor Banks, University of Massachusetts Medical Center, 55 Lake Avenue North, Worcester, Massachusetts 01655. The telephone number is (508) 756-6444.

THE HMO PATIENT

ᣮ

If you are being treated at an HMO (Health Maintenance Organization), bear in mind that by their very nature, HMOs are not geared to do the necessary *staging* of the disease or to treat unusual cancers aggressively. Staging is the breakdown into categories indicating the spread of the disease. Staging a cancer involves extensive scans, X-rays, laboratory tests and other specific diagnostic procedures to determine if the cancer has spread and if so, to what extent. The staging of a cancer is what usually determines what the state-of-art treatment would be.

I recommend to my Medicare clients who belong to an HMO that they drop the HMO and switch back to Medicare, which will cover most of a patient's cancer treatment costs. The value of being on Medicare is that it does not limit you in your choice of a physician or a hospital. Yet it is amazing how many patients are reluctant to change their medical insurance even though they know they may not get the best or the most aggressive treatment at the HMO.

The Mayo Comprehensive Cancer Center program provides consultations to HMOs, so if you live in that vicinity you can obtain a second opinion, a confirmation of diagnosis and other services that can make a big difference, especially if you have a complicated cancer.

FINDING SPECIAL RESOURCES

For a patient whose cancer seems to evade all treatment, it can be overwhelmingly disappointing to find out that you are not a trial candidate, but you can do two things with the disappointment. You can keep looking; new things come up all the time. You might want to explore a non-toxic therapy or alternative cancer treatment (see Chapter 17), or you may seek conventional therapies in the hands of innovative physicians.

In your quest, the potential for disappointment is immense, but so is the possible gain. In search of that gain, I often refer cancer patients to Dr. Isaac Djerassi at the Cancer Mini-Center he developed at Mercy Catholic Medical Center Misericordia Hospital in Philadelphia.

Dr. Djerassi is the pioneer of high-dose methotrexate (see Chapter 8) and developed a rescue technique to counteract the many serious side effects of the drug. The high doses necessary to affect the tumor require a leucovorin *rescue*. The purpose of the technique is simple but vitally important. Citrovorum factor, also known as leucovorin *rescue*, is administered at prescribed intervals to counteract or protect the patient from the harmful effects of high-dose methotrexate, which can be life threatening. This rescue technique is very exacting, and slip-ups on the part of the doctor could have devastating effects on the patient.

I stayed for three weeks with a patient and his family at Dr. Djerassi's Cancer Mini-Center, Philadelphia. In the course of those weeks, I had the opportunity to speak to many of the patients and their families, and we discussed numerous aspects of their disease. I learned about the remarkable research capabilities of Dr. Djerassi and observed his clinical applications. I was impressed with his subtle modifications of treatment of each patient.

I often recommend a consultation with him when a patient has a tumor that might respond to methotrexate, though his approach is not limited to methotrexate. I have seen patients of his who have been treated with a whole gamut of anti-cancer drugs as well as immunotherapy, as was mentioned in Chapter 6.

In many cases, Dr. Djerassi has told a patient, "You are getting the best treatment where you are. I don't have anything better to offer." But I also know of other times when, after learning the details of a case, he's responded with enthusiastic excitement, "Can you come right away? I'll have a bed waiting for you. I think I can help."

In the course of my work, I have met several cancer patients who were treated by or consulted with Dr. Rudy Falk at the Falk Oncology Centre, Ltd. This address is 890 Yonge Street, 2nd Floor, Toronto, Ontario, M4W IP3, Canada. The telephone number is (416) 921-2525. Many cancer patients who have not responded to standard treatments find their way to Dr. Falk, who is known as a developer of innovative therapies. In addition to directing his own center, Dr. Falk is Surgical Oncologist at the Toronto General Hospital. He offers hope to patients who have been told, "There is nothing more that can be done."

At the Centre, mobilization of the immune system is emphasized. Non-steroidal anti-inflammatory drugs (NSAIDS) are used in combination with a carrier molecule, hyaluronic acid. The NSAIDS provide the mechanism to block the overproduction of excessive prostaglandins (a body chemical) which in turn allows the macrophages (scavenger cells), which are the body's first line in the immune defense system, to be activated. High doses of vitamin C combined with hyaluronic acid are also administered to act as antioxidants (free-radical scavengers). Other anti-cancer agents and methods are used such as regional hyperthermia and chemotherapy. Chemotherapy administered is at much lower than standard doses and once again is combined with the carrier molecule which helps the chemotherapy target the abnormal tissue and carry it across the cell membrane.

When used in conjunction with this approach, lower doses of conventional treatments, such as radiation and chemotherapy, can be effective. The patient is not subjected to the possible painful side effects of high doses of chemotherapy, and there is less weakening of the immune system. This in turn enhances the quality of life for patients. Treatment is given on an outpatient basis, and the costs are covered by most insurance companies.

There are other pioneering specialists out there. As I've mentioned, recovered cancer patients can be an excellent source of this information. Results from research and investigative trials abound, and the professional and lay media report them all the time. But be careful about getting your hopes up from every bit of cancer news you hear or read about. I checked out several news articles on promising studies only to find that the research reported was still in laboratory trials, was no longer relevant, or was many years away from being available as a treatment.

I first heard of Stanislaw Burzynski, M.D., Ph.D., of the Burzynski Research Institute in Texas from several grateful patients. His early research was at Baylor College of Medicine with partial funding from the National Cancer Institute.

In the treatment of cancer, Dr. Burzynski uses Antineoplastons, *messenger* peptides, which are biochemicals in the body that interact with DNA. When a cell's DNA is damaged, the resulting misinformation can lead to abnormal cell development or cancer. According to Dr. Burzynski's research, our body can normalize these potential cancer cells through these *messenger* peptides which bond to cancer cells, feeding them the complex information they need to fulfill their original function. Dr. Burzynski has found that there is a marked deficiency of these peptides in cancer patients.

The Antineoplastons are non-toxic and are able to penetrate the blood brain barrier (a system that allows only certain chemicals to enter the brain). This approach has proven most successful with brain tumors, prostate cancers and lymphomas. They are given by mouth in capsule form or are injected. Treatment can last from nine months to two years depending upon the type and intensity of the disease.

The Institute is at 6221 Corporate Drive, Houston, Texas 77036; telephone: (713) 777-8233.

In December, 1991, the Institute announced that the National Cancer Institute plans to conduct four independent Phase II trials in brain tumors using Antineoplastons. A call to the CIS will keep you posted on the outcome.

You never know where you will find someone able to help you. In 1987, Ann Landers, acting on a tip from a reader, investigated a doctor in Quebec who reputedly had developed a highly successful treatment for prostate cancer. Using her very thorough research methods, she found that Dr. Fernand Labrie was indeed on to something. Using a hormonal approach instead of the very traumatic standard treatment, castration, he achieved remission in all 87 of the patients who had come to him before getting other treatments. Unfortunately, few of those who had any previous treatment improved. This demonstrates why it is critical to research your case before you start any treatment.

Ann Landers wanted to know why this treatment was available only in Canada. She found out from the National Cancer Institute that one of the two drugs Dr. Labrie was using had not been approved by the Food and Drug Administration.

In July, 1987, my own research turned up Dr. Norman L. Block of the University of Miami Sylvester Comprehensive Cancer Center who reported the availability of LHRH hormone treatment for advanced prostate cancer. This treatment decreases the production of male hormones which increase the activity of prostate cancer. Hormonal treatments are now standard protocol for prostate cancers that have spread.

Dr. Labrie's treatment includes a second hormone, Flutamide (Eulexin), which is taken orally in addition to the LHRH hormone, and it is used on early cancers also. Mind you, this is no panacea as the use of the hormones causes infertility, and after long-term use, patients can become resistant to the hormones. This treatment requires continued use of pills and daily or monthly injections. Thus, an active man might not want to be tied down to daily or monthly office visits to his doctor for LHRH injections whereas a man in his eighties might prefer this course of treatment rather than surgery. The important point is that the patient be given a choice so he can elect the treatment that is most tolerable for him.

In any case, it is important to take the antiandrogen (antihormonal agent) in order to block the male hormones originating from the adrenals and which remain free to stimulate prostate cancer after castration. Dr. Labrie is at the Centre de Recherche du Chul, Centre Hospitalier de l'Université Laval, 2705 Boul. Laurier, Québec, G1V 4G2, Canada; telephone (418) 654-2244.

In the course of my research, I found a number of breast cancer patients and one prostate cancer patient who developed *lymphedema* and who had not been cautioned about how to try to avert getting the condition and when they did, how to get proper care for it. Some patients who have had radiation therapy or have had lymph nodes removed suffer from chronic swelling of an arm or leg. Sometimes immobility of the limb develops also. This condition is called lymphedema and results from damage to or obstruction of the lymph nodes and vessels. As fluid becomes trapped in the space between cells, the swelling increases, and a limb can become disfigured. Special pumps (sequential gradient pumps), massage (manual lymph drainage), and compression stockings and sleeves can be used to reduce the swelling.

If lymphedema is not treated, it can lead to severe complications. A very informative pamphlet is available to assist with information about the causes, symptoms, and treatment of lymphedema, how it can be prevented, and ways to deal with this complication of cancer therapy. To obtain a list of Lymphedema Treatment Centers and Manual Lymph Drainage Therapists and the informational pamphlet, write or call The National Lymphedema Network, 2211 Post Street, Suite 404, San Francisco, California 94115. The telephone number 1-800-541-3259.

HOME INFUSION THERAPIES

 है

For some patients, it is a great boon to be able to receive chemotherapy at home. Some treatment protocols call for slow continuous infusion of anti-cancer agents. Patients with certain types of cancer have been found to benefit from this type of home chemotherapy infusion. In addition to convenience, this service can enhance the comfort and state of mind of patients and can reduce costs of patient management as well.

Sometimes cancer patients are temporarily unable to swallow and may have internal nutrition therapy prescribed, but only when the patient can digest the nutritional formula.

Cancer patients diagnosed with malnutrition are prime candidates for total peritoneal nutrition (TPN), also referred to as hyperalimentation. This is a mixture that, depending upon the patient's medical needs, is comprised of specific amounts of proteins, carbohydrates, fats, vitamins and minerals, electrolytes and water required by the patient.

Such home infusion therapies are available through Home Nursing Service (HNS) centers located throughout the country. The national office is in Pine Brook, New Jersey. If you call 1-800-872-4467, you will be connected to the service center nearest you. I was told they could arrange these services for patients in most outlying or rural areas through their closest service center. They report a 24-hour on-call IV team, pharmacy services, and warehouse and delivery, as well as a round-the-clock patient hot line.

HNS is accredited by the Joint Commission on the Accreditation of Healthcare Organizations (JCAHO).

An article in the business section of a local newspaper led me to Home Intensive Care, Inc. in North Miami Beach, which I learned was another qualified national provider of these home health-care services. They have service centers at 27 operating locations in 45 geographic areas and are accredited by CHAP (Community Health Accreditation Program) which is a subsidiary of the National League of Nursing. Corporate headquarters are at 150 Northwest 168th Street, Miami Beach, Florida 33169. They can be contacted at 1-800-344-3181.

There are other comparable providers of services such as these. Ask your physician or the social services department at your hospital for a referral.

Sometimes, the decision against journeying to a distant center may grow out of denial. The patient may be using this decision to deny the seriousness of the condition. It may seem that by simply seeing a local doctor the patient can still believe: I'm not so sick. This can't be so deadly if a local doctor can treat me.

In fact, the effort of getting a second opinion at a distant medical center may create a sense of urgency which may be more than the patient believes he or she can handle. If the sense of urgency, or the extra effort is threatening to you, try to turn it around and make it work. You might tell yourself, Sure, I know this is urgent. Cancer demands a sense of urgency. I'm going to waste no time getting the best treatment I can find or afford so I can put this behind me.

PROFILE OF AN ONCOLOGIST —
FINDING THE BEST

Satisfy yourself that you have researched your case as carefully, as completely, as possible. After all, the first rule of warfare is to understand your enemy. What follows is an example of the type of physician who you can be sure can help or can direct you to whom to see, what to do, and where to go.

In the previous chapter, I wrote about Dr. Edward J. Beattie. I first heard of him when he was Chief of Surgery at Jackson Memorial Hospital in Miami. He came to Jackson from Memorial Sloan-Kettering Cancer Center where one of his many positions was Chief Medical Officer. He is presently director of the Kriser Lung Cancer Center at Beth Israel Hospital in New York City, as well as its Chief of Thoracic Surgery. He is Professor of Surgery at Mount Sinai Hospital and Doctors Hospital, director of cancer activities at Beth Israel Medical Center, all in New York City, and is a surgical consultant to Rockefeller Hospital.

Dr. Beattie reports having access to residents and to fellows that he trained in Chicago and at Memorial Sloan-Kettering. Memorial has an alumni directory of the hundreds of fellows trained at their institute. Dr. Beattie maintains close connections with oncologists and former trainees in the United States and around the world, including Bombay and Japan, to whom he can refer patients.

When he treats patients, he considers himself part of a team that includes local doctors, with whom he works closely, and when he turns the patient back over to them, he says, "I tell them what we found, what we did, and what we plan."

Dr. Beattie's philosophy is, "You are our patient for life. Patients become our friends." He works with the whole family. He works on building bridges and friendships. This is the quality of physicians found at top cancer centers.

... PERSONAL PERSPECTIVE

ટ✍

In this chapter, I've thrown out a lot of heavy material in terms of where you might go and what you might do. I know it's not always easy to do this. I suffered many agonies in my search for the best treatment. Each call to a physician, and there were many, was difficult — preparing my questions, keeping the doctors on the phone long enough to get my answers, asking for clarification, then discovering after hanging up and digesting the material that I had new questions. The doctors' annoyance with further calls was almost more than I could bear. I might have wept a bit in anticipation of difficulty, but invariably I would pull myself together and make the call again.

As discussed earlier, studies show that more aggressive patients have longer rates of survival than do their passive counterparts. Telling yourself, "I'm worth it!" leads you to take charge of your own case and to become an aggressive patient.

Chapter 10

THE PATIENT'S PLEDGE:
HOW TO MAKE MEDICAL PROFESSIONALS
WANT TO MEET YOUR NEEDS

As a patient, you need to assert yourself to make sure that your doctors and the hospital provide the kind of high-quality care you need. Don't be intimidated. Most hospitals are staffed with capable, caring but beleaguered people; appreciate them, but appreciate yourself, too.

A hospital represents both comfort and threat. The comfort comes from the sense of protection offered by routine, from the very size of the institution, which seems to speak of vast knowledge and resources, as well as the warmth, experience, compassion and support of many of the people who work within it. But patients also feel threatened by the unknown. You'd be surprised at the number of otherwise well-adjusted adults who don't feel comfortable in a hospital — even as visitors. It's not just the institutional environment or the whiff of disinfectant in the air. The hospital reminds us that health, which is often taken for granted, is not a given.

That feeling of discomfort is magnified when you're a patient. It's easy to become as passive mentally as you are physically. Your normal life has been interrupted. You are in an unfamiliar room in an unfamiliar bed, at the foot of which hangs an indecipherable chart, which regulates your new, incomprehensible life. Even your meals are served on someone else's schedule from someone else's menu.

You don't feel well and you're scared.

There are two easy *outs*, and you shouldn't take either of them. One is a sense of benign acceptance, which can lead one to being controlled or managed. The other is fright induced by insistent waves of paranoia, which can lead to hostility and a failure to communicate.

As a patient, you must stay alert, ask questions and become a respected active partner in your own healing process.

It's not easy, but it is worth doing.

To become active in your own behalf, you need to inaugurate your personal Patient's Pledge:

THE PATIENT'S PLEDGE

Rule 1:   I will be heard.
Rule 2:   I will not be intimidated.
Rule 3:   I will listen to my body; my symptoms matter.
Rule 4:   I will be fully informed and be included in the final decision.
Rule 5:   I will have the best care.
Rule 6:   I am entitled to hope.
Rule 7:   I am entitled to compassion and to be treated with dignity.
Rule 8:   I will stand up for my own best interests.
Rule 9:   I will praise good care and report bad care.
Rule 10: I will be safe.

RULE 1: I WILL BE HEARD

Many patients, especially those who are loners with virtually no family or friends from whom to derive support, are afraid to make waves. They don't assert themselves because they don't want trouble. They are afraid that if they called their doctors too many times about their pain or asked a nurse to give some small attention to their comfort, they might not help them when they need them even more.

Ironically, patients' submissive behavior may help bring about the very situation they fear most. Because they don't speak up for themselves and have no one to speak up for them, they simply aren't heard. And when the pain of their condition gets so out of control that they can no longer contain themselves, they present their problems in a highly emotional state. Their doctors and nurses often respond to their emotional state and do not hear what the patients are trying to tell them about their bodies.

This can set off a chain reaction of misunderstandings, which can undermine patients' health even more.

Psychologist and cellular biologist Joan Borysenko found that patients who accept whatever the doctors tell them and have trouble expressing any emotions at all apparently don't have as much of a chance against cancer. They just don't put up a fight. On the other hand, she notes, "The cancer survivors are often feisty complainers. They're tagged as difficult patients to work with because they may not comply very readily." They ask, "Why are you doing this to me? What are my choices?"

It may take several trips to the front line to train yourself to be a good soldier in your own battle. You must learn to assert yourself. You must train yourself to put your emotions on hold and to let your intellect be in charge. You must practice what you want to say and how you want to say it, so you will be ready to act when necessary.

* * * * *

*I exercised Rule 1 (*I Will Be Heard*) when my doctor ignored a request I made. Because I had had an allergic reaction to one of the chemotherapies at Dana-Farber, my oncologist, Dr. Arthur Skarin put me on an antihistamine (Benadryl) before the infusion. When I returned home to complete my chemotherapy, Dr. Skarin referred me to an oncologist in Florida. The new oncologist wanted to include adrenalin before my infusion as a precautionary measure, and he insisted on my being in intensive care for*

24 hours afterwards. That sounded okay to me. I'm all for taking precautions.

During one of my trips to intensive care, my doctor's associate, who was covering for him, made further changes in the protocol. He added an additional medication without telling me what it was or what it was expected to accomplish. I refused to take it. I continued to refuse, "Unless," I told him, "you tell me what new medication you ordered." He finally relented and told me it was cortisone. I asked him why I needed that. His answer was, "As an added precaution." I already had plenty of cortisone in my other chemotherapy protocol, and cortisone can have significant side effects. So I told him, "No, thanks, I'll pass. I don't care to take more cortisone just to be more cautious."

Unfortunately, I had to repeat myself several times before my message got through. But I stuck to my firm no-nonsense tone of voice until I was heard. This is not to say it was easy. I had all kinds of knots in my stomach while I went through that scenario, but when the doctor finally agreed not to include the cortisone, I felt better.

RULE 2: I WILL NOT BE INTIMIDATED

Too often, doctors manipulate their patients subtly by responding to their questions or complaints with, "Well, I don't see anything wrong." Patients who persist in describing how awful they feel sometimes hear, "Maybe you ought to be treated elsewhere." A patient who questions the doctor's treatment recommendations may even be told, "If that's the way you feel, perhaps you should find someone else to treat you."

What the patient hears — in all these messages (even when they come from sincere doctors who convey them unwittingly by not responding or by a sharp tone of voice) — is a thinly veiled threat: "If you act up or make too many demands, I don't want to treat you anymore."

Patients tend to fall into the trap, thinking, "Oh, no, who will I go to now? I'll have to start all over with someone.

If my doctor won't see me, what will I do?" Such patients become compliant wimps. While some doctors may prefer a patient who tucks away symptoms and fears, that's not the doctor for you.

Many of you are afraid to change doctors. So, you stay with the doctor you know, no matter what your doubts are. You're not alone in this dilemma. Doctors or their families who become ill with cancer have the same problem and often sacrifice quality care on the altar of loyalty. They don't want to hurt a colleague's feelings. I knew one doctor who had lung cancer. His office was across the street from a cancer center where an outstanding lung cancer specialist practiced. Yet, when I mentioned this to him, he shook his head. "Oh, I'm being treated by a colleague of mine. I'm in good hands," he said.

The fear of their doctors that cancer patients feel is one of the most difficult things I grapple with as a therapist. I urge them to speak up; if the physicians are good, they'll be appreciated.

The worst that can happen is that your doctor will no longer see you. If this happens, get out your *so what* tape. Getting a new physician on your case may be the best thing that could happen to you. Intimidation is a trap — sometimes we set it ourselves; sometimes our doctors or nurses set it. Either way, we can always refuse to fall in.

* * * * *

Almost a year had passed since I had been in remission and I still felt weak. Surely I ought to feel a little better. Was I really just overanxious? Perhaps not . . .

I wanted answers, so I made an appointment with an oncologist at an outstanding cancer center. At my second check-up, I told him about the pain — in my throat.

"I don't see anything there," he told me after he peered into my throat.

"I'm worried because my throat felt just like this a year and a half ago," I told him. "My doctors couldn't see anything then either until it nearly choked me."

He answered curtly, "Come back in four months." I

was flabbergasted. My New York doctors instructed me to be followed up every two months for two years. He knew that. It was in my records. His behavior sent me a very negative message. After this ugly, shattering experience, I never went back to him.

While I was floundering, my pharmacist recommended another oncologist. Pharmacists are excellent sources of information on doctors. They often know which ones patients complain about and those who are helping people effectively.

I made an appointment with the new oncologist, the late Dr. Jacob Colsky. He asked me for a detailed history of my medical condition; he was kindly; he didn't rush me; and he took concrete steps to check out my symptoms.

I could have cried with relief. At last, someone was listening! But it only came to pass because I was not intimidated by my previous doctor into behaving like a compliant wimp. When he didn't address my complaints, I found a doctor who did.

RULE 3: I WILL LISTEN TO MY BODY; MY SYMPTOMS MATTER

No one knows what's going on in your body as well as you do. Your job as a patient is to relay your body's messages to your physician, so he or she can get an accurate picture of your condition. That important process begins in the physician's office, at the moment of your first contact. Few people are comfortable in a doctor's office. The stress and fear you may feel make it hard to communicate effectively, so it's important to spend some time getting prepared in advance.

Many patients, especially the isolated ones, bring in so much personal and family history that the doctor needs to tune out such conversation to hone in on the primary medical complaint. All the extra information can make it difficult for the physician to define and treat actual physical problems.

Before your first appointment, take your own history. Be specific. Jot down all the relevant points — symptoms, suspicions, past treatments. State how long you've been having these symptoms — one week, two weeks, a month — how often the pain occurs — all day, six or seven times a day, every few days, or only after meals — and how severe it is. To be accurate about the severity of a symptom like pain or bleeding, it helps to keep track of it on a scale of one to ten. For example, one for the least amount and ten for the most severe. Create your own picture of your condition, preparing your case carefully so your physician can see it clearly.

It is also important to remember everything the doctor tells you. You might want to take notes, bring a friend or relative to help you keep track, or even tape-record the physician's instructions.

* * * * *

A little more than six months after my last radiation treatment, I felt more listless and tired than ever. I continually reported my low energy to my oncologist. He kept telling me, "Everything looks fine. It just takes time." I couldn't shake the constant sluggishness, I was gaining weight and getting puffy around the face, and my thinking wasn't clear.

While looking at the family photos we took at my son's high school graduation, I was struck by my resemblance to an old biology textbook's picture of a woman with myxedema (underactive thyroid) or hypothyroidism. Suddenly, everything clicked. I had had two-thirds of my thyroid removed at the time of my surgery. My doctor in New York told me he would instruct my oncologist in Miami to follow up on my thyroid function. My Miami oncologist never did.

"Doctor," I asked my oncologist, "don't you think I should have a thyroid test?"

"Oh, sure," he answered casually. When the results came back, I registered a 2 when the normal range was 6-10. I had hypothyroidism. The physician put me on synthroid, a thyroid medication, and I immediately improved.

RULE 4: I WILL BE
FULLY INFORMED
ॐ

Be honest with yourself. If you don't understand something your physician says, don't be proud or shy. Stop. Ask for an explanation or a definition. You can't act in your own behalf unless you understand what the doctor is telling you. Most people don't understand medical terms. If you need an unfamiliar word or phrase explained, ask your doctor to re-phrase his thought in lay language. Remember, your doctor went to medical school, you didn't! This is the time, before surgery or a biopsy, to ask about preserving tissue in special ways for possible tests later in the course of your treatment. It is also the time to learn whether there are alternative courses of treatment. You want to learn about all your options. Be sure you make that clear to the physician.

Don't be shy about pulling out a list of questions in front of your physician. After all, nobody thinks anything of taking a list to the grocery store. When it comes to pleasing your taste buds, you don't want to forget a single treat. It's much more crucial to remember everything that might help your physician evaluate your condition.

Question the experience of the physician that will do special diagnostic tests. You need qualified specialists with special training to perform these procedures and to correctly interpret the results.

* * * * *

When your physician makes his treatment recommendation, ask:

* Upon what are his decisions based? His intuition? Medical tests? On the stage of the disease? If so, what stage is it in?

* What tests were done to determine the stage of my disease? Are there any other tests that might have been done but weren't? If so, why not?

* Is this standard treatment for that stage? Are there any other treatments for this stage?

* Are there any investigational trials for this stage? Would you recommend an investigational trial at this point? If yes, why? What are the risks and/or the benefits? What are the chances for remission? Cure? If this is an investigational trial, how many patients have you treated with this protocol? How many went into remission? How many were cured? How many died?

* What are the credentials of the laboratory that diagnosed the disease? Is this an HMO laboratory or one in a general hospital that doesn't diagnose or treat many cancer patients each year? If so, tell him you would feel better with a second interpretation at a laboratory at a Comprehensive or Clinical Cancer Center, or one such as was mentioned in Chapter 6.

* Could I benefit from being treated at a CCC or a Medical Center with more expertise in treating this condition? If the answer is no, ask why not.

* Are there any tests that can predict the potential of my tumor to spread or to be aggressive?

* If either radiation therapy or chemotherapy is recommended, what are the pros and cons of each? Which is more aggressive? Which suppresses the immune system more? What would you go with if this were you? Why? Is your decision a medical one or is it based on quality of life or any other factors?

* I understood that surgery and radiation destroy cancer cells in the tumor and some of the surrounding area only, and that chemotherapy travels throughout the body to destroy malignant cells. With this in mind, if I have surgery and/or radiation or radiation alone—would it be advisable to have chemotherapy as a preventive measure to destroy any cancer cells that may break off and spread to some far off site?

* If I go with the treatment you recommend, will that rule me out as a candidate for another approach at a later date should I need it? If so, would I have other options?

* Is this an aggressive approach that you are recommending? If not, why? I've heard with cancer you need the biggest blast first time around to get on top of the disease.

* What are the chances of my disease recurring? If

they are high, are you recommending an aggressive approach? If not, why?

* Are there any alternative therapies that you know of that have been known to have a measure of success with my disease?

* Is there anything about my diagnosis or your treatment plan or the expected outcome that I should know that I haven't asked?

This line of questioning shouldn't take more than ten or fifteen minutes and with a disease as serious as cancer, you're entitled to that much time to discuss your concerns. If you are not satisfied with your doctor's reactions to your questions, and certainly if you are uncomfortable with his ability to reply, as I have said repeatedly, he is obviously not the doctor for you.

If, on the other hand, you feel confident he has responded to all your concerns with knowledgeable answers, I suggest you tell him, "I feel comfortable, doctor, with your competence, and I appreciate your relating to all my needs. I want you to direct my treatment. But, before we begin, I would like a second opinion from a specialist who is not affiliated with you."

* * * * *

My initial introduction into the cancer scene came about when my ear, nose and throat doctor told me that my thyroid was palpable *and ordered a thyroid scan. I was too embarrassed by my own ignorance to admit I didn't know what* palpable *meant, so I didn't ask. I didn't learn until a year later that* palpable *meant that he could feel a growth in my throat . . . a lump. Had I inquired at the time and learned what* palpable *meant, I would have been more alarmed and probably more active in my own behalf.*

But responsibility between doctor and patient is a two-way street. Had my doctor made sure that I understood what he had told me and explored the possibility of other tests, maybe my cancer would have been detected at an earlier and more treatable stage.

RULE 5: I WILL HAVE
THE BEST CARE

ट्~

You can't just hope for the best. You have to demand it and seek it. You need to be assured that you are getting the most competent care possible.

Shortly after former President Reagan's colon surgery in 1985, several reputable specialists publicly questioned the quality of the treatment he received. After Mrs. Reagan had a mastectomy, other doctors asked if such radical surgery was necessary. If the Chief Executive and the First Lady can't get medical care that is beyond question — how can you? The answer is by being alert, asking questions, asking other experts and exerting yourself until you have established to your own complete satisfaction that you've chosen the right professional.

What if your car was out of whack and your regular mechanic couldn't fix it? You wouldn't hesitate to take it to another garage. Shouldn't you be at least as determined when your body isn't working?

You can learn a lot from the physician's behavior. A good doctor listens. He pays attention to what you are saying as carefully as he examines your body. Often, clues culled from the patient's history or little things that crop up from visit to visit can help the doctor order the right tests and make the right diagnosis.

Nobody knows whether you are hurting or what you are feeling unless you communicate it to them. But communication also involves listening. Most physicians listen, and most are caring and competent. But there are incompetent practitioners in every profession, including the medical profession. Protect yourself from the bad apples.

* * * * *

I'm grateful to Dr. Moses Nussbaum at Beth Israel Hospital in New York City for a very special consideration. The evening before my scheduled biopsy, a student nurse appeared in my room and told me that my doctor had requested a nurse in training be assigned to be with me

*before, during and after the surgery. She spoke to me about
the operation and what I could expect. She explained that
she would be in my room in the morning to help me with my
shower or with whatever else I needed and would be with
me in the operating room and the recovery room as well. She
was very helpful and kept me so occupied that my scary
thoughts didn't have a chance to overwhelm my mind. How
nice I thought. It didn't occur to me until much later that the
doctor must have anticipated the possibility of a dire
outcome to the surgery to make such an unusual request. I
am thankful the surgery went well and can still remember
how good it felt to have that student nurse wrap me in
heated blankets in the recovery room when my body couldn't
stop shaking from the cold that I felt. It was also comforting
to have someone there to hold my hand.*

*It's doctors like Dr. Nussbaum who, in addition to
their expertise, want only the best for their patients and they
see to it that they get it.*

RULE 6: I AM ENTITLED TO HOPE

As a patient, you'll soon become aware that one of the
most sensitive moments in your relationship with your
physician is when he delivers your prognosis. The words he
uses are so important.

I'm all for physicians being frank with their patients.
But I take issue with any doctor who acts as the self-
appointed angel of death and *sentences* a patient to a
certain number of weeks or months. That physician is
robbing a human being of the last vestiges of hope.

No physician, however skilled, is a licensed prophet.
Doctors are trained to heal. When they say there is nothing
more that can be done, they are actually saying that there
is nothing more they personally can do. That's an important distinction. When you hear these negatives pro-
nounced with finality, it's wise to find another doctor.

* * * * *

There is also something else that could be tried, such as the little-understood rallying power of prayer, or the eternal energy of looking toward the future.

I often recommend patients go to a comprehensive cancer center for a second opinion. After their visit, I repeatedly hear patients say, "I can't thank you enough, Sarah, for telling me about the cancer center. The doctor was great. He was kind. He didn't rush me. He answered all my questions. He explained what he would do and everything I could expect. He seemed confident and sure and very knowledgeable. And he's going to have me go before a whole team of experts who will review my case."

"It's scary but he's assured me he's done many surgeries of this type. His confidence is reassuring. I came away from there full of hope."

This is how I felt every time I walked through the swinging doors of Dana-Farber Cancer Institute when I was being treated there.

RULE 7: I AM ENTITLED TO COMPASSION AND TO BE TREATED WITH DIGNITY

Sometimes physicians and other health care workers may be unintentionally callous in their treatment of a patient. Their work becomes so routine they forget they are dealing with vulnerable human beings. Another common hazard among professionals dedicated to serving critically ill people is that many of them develop some sense of distance to keep from being constantly depressed. But a protective, professional attitude doesn't excuse callous behavior.

For the sake of many patients who are subjected to life support or treatments for which they were never consulted, on December 1, 1991, the Patient Self-Determination Act went into effect. This requires hospitals and other medical facilities to inform patients at the time of admission of their right to refuse treatment or to have life support turned off. At the same time Medicare and Medicaid patients will be asked if they have a document that spells out their wishes regarding resuscitation or other extraordinary means of preserving life in the event they are unable to make decisions for themselves. This is an important turn of events. Patients are better able to make a decision of this magnitude seated at a desk in the admissions office (or they can ask for a little time to think about it and get back with an answer) than when in an intensive care unit or when in critical condition in their hospital bed.

For some people, a question like, "Do you wish to be placed on life support?" when they are near death might, in fact, hasten death.

A wise patient can execute a Durable Power of Attorney or in states where applicable a Living Will. The Durable Power of Attorney document allows you to appoint someone to make decisions about your health care and/or whatever else you specify. It is reversible or can be changed at any time. A Living Will specifies what you would like done if you have a medical emergency and are unable to make decisions. Painful as these matters may be for some to think about, if you don't specify what are your wishes in case you can't make a decision and there is an emergency, your doctor makes it for you. And that is usually a medical decision.

You will have peace of mind knowing you made clear whom you want to make decisions for you if the need should arise. Many patients feel good about doing this as it assures them they are still in control of the events of their lives. The CIS can give you information about Durable Power of Attorney and Living Wills in your state.

Once, when I was in intensive care for chemotherapy, a resident very casually started poking my arm in search of a vein to start the IV. I asked the young physician to be more careful. "No problem," said he. "When these go, we can always get veins in your toes or your head." In a well-modulated, assertive tone which I used to convey the dignity I was demanding from him, I said: "Doctor, I'm in enough pain already. I can't handle you telling me about IVs in my head or my toes. I expect you to treat my veins carefully. If you can't, perhaps it would be better if we asked someone else to insert this IV."

Don't suffer in silence. Let your doctor know immediately what he is doing that offends you.

Another case in point is that of a woman who told me how degraded she felt when a young resident came into her hospital room to examine her. He poked and prodded. He lifted her gown to examine her breasts, then continued the rest of his examination. He left her gown open and her body was exposed during the entire time. She told me in a very painful voice, "I felt like a hunk of flesh. It was awful."

I make it a point to cover the parts of my body that the doctor is not examining. If a physician doesn't afford us that dignity, we need to give it to ourselves.

* * * * *

When it was time to go to Boston for my first methotrexate treatment, I was terribly frightened. Methotrexate involved so many warnings and directions. Unfortunately, Seymore couldn't be with me on this trip, so I would have to manage everything alone.

I was full of trepidation as I read and reread my instruction sheet the evening before I was to leave Miami. I felt a little uneasy doing it, but when my fears mounted, I called Dr. Mayer, Chief of the Adult Clinic, Dana-Farber Cancer Institute at home. Dr. Robert Mayer and Dr. Arthur Skarin, my primary physician, had given me their home telephone numbers, but I hated to disturb them. When I apologized for calling the doctor at home, he warmly assured me that he didn't mind at all. He said it was perfectly all right.

I told him of my concern about the methotrexate and thought I'd feel better if I could check into the hospital. Dr. Mayer took time to convince me that I'd be fine. The clinic was close to the house. If I needed anything, I could call a special 24-hour hot line. He was very reassuring. Although I was still not totally at ease, I understood it would be okay to get my treatment as an out-patient.

The compassion of outstanding doctors such as Dr.

Mayer, Dr. Skarin, Dr. Frei and others like them was more than gratifying, and I think their concern, personal interest and confidence was an important factor in my belief that I would survive.

RULE 8: I WILL STAND UP FOR MY OWN BEST INTERESTS

Of all the professionals you'll deal with, you are likely to have the most interaction with nurses. For the most part, the nurses who look after you will treat you well. They will be genuine, caring people, devoted to their work. When I was in intensive care, I observed how hard the specially-trained nurses in that unit worked and was impressed and heartened by their dedication and kindness.

Special attentions happen in places where the patient is the first concern. But when routine is king, the patient has to be assertive. You must stand up for yourself if you're being wronged. Too many patients back down as soon as they meet resistance from a doctor or nurse.

I once saw a skinny, bald little boy, about six years old, cringing and squirming on the floor of the blood lab in a hospital. His mother was trying unsuccessfully to pick him up so that a nurse could draw blood from his vein. My heart went out to him. I couldn't help myself; I intervened. I gently told the mother that — if this was for a blood count — she could get the doctor's permission to have the sample drawn from a finger prick. I explained that I had just done that myself. She looked startled. "Oh, no, I couldn't do that," she said, "I couldn't bother the doctor." She had more concern for how the doctor would react to her request than to what was best for her son.

Promise yourself to stand up for your own best interests; if your assertiveness falters, think of that poor little boy.

* * * * *

I'm especially indebted to the nurses in the Dana-Farber blood lab for teaching me an important lesson about looking out for my welfare. A regular part of my scheduled visits was a blood test — taken from a finger prick, not directly from a vein. The nurses explained that this method saved my veins for the intravenous chemotherapy and IV's I needed in the course of my long-term treatment. Overused veins have a tendency to collapse. Chemotherapy can wreak havoc on them.

Blood results are more accurate when taken from blood from a vein, but if you are going to need numerous blood counts during the course of your chemotherapy, check with your doctor. He may agree that it may be more important in the course of your cancer therapy to spare your veins whenever possible. Your doctor can always order a count from blood taken from a vein if it proves to be necessary.

I made seven trips to intensive care for one of the chemotherapies. At that hospital, blood counts were routinely obtained from blood drawn from a vein. I discussed having this done from a finger prick with my oncologist before I was admitted to the hospital. He thought it was a good idea and agreed to order my blood counts to be taken from a finger prick. The technicians didn't like it. The blood lab didn't like it. But I stood my ground. The hospital and health care professionals were there to serve my best interests. I intended to see that they did.

RULE 9: I WILL PRAISE GOOD CARE AND REPORT BAD CARE

Vindictive nurses and surly orderlies should not be tolerated. The management of the hospital wants you to get quality care. In most hospitals, nurses and technicians depend on good reports in frequent reviews to keep their jobs and to qualify for advancement. Patients must report abusive behavior. If you feel unequal to the task, enlist someone close to you.

This approach applies to non-medical service personnel and technicians also. These service people are often compassionate and well-trained. But if you encounter someone rude and unpleasant, take action.

* * * * *

At one time, my tests included bone marrow aspiration, which can be an excruciatingly painful procedure. At each step of the way, my doctor told me what to expect. He could not have been more caring. But I'll never forget that day. The doctor was almost finished when I heard a rude voice boom through the curtains and demand to cart me off immediately to my next test, a liver scan.

"You'll have to wait," my physician said, "we're not quite done here." I heard a grumbled response that urged the doctor to hurry.

As the doctor completed the procedure and pulled open the curtains around my bed, I gingerly lifted myself up. When the young man from the transport service who was waiting with a wheelchair saw me, he snorted. He was really ticked off that I held him up and that I still needed a few minutes to compose myself. I had to allow myself the dignity to apply some lipstick, find my book, and pick up a sweater to wear in the chilly corridors.

Once I deposited myself in the wheelchair, the young man's behavior became monstrous. He pushed me roughly through the corridors, cussing: "Do you know how many people you're holding up? Who do you think you are?" On and on, until I was ready to scream.

"Hold it, young man," I said at last, as I painfully raised myself out of the wheelchair. "I'm not going any further with you." Shaken and exhausted, I walked haltingly back to my room and reported the incident to the transport and scanning departments and to the nurse supervisor. I didn't have my liver scan that day, but I made my point. Unfortunately, that satisfaction didn't take away the emotional trauma . . . but it helped lessen it.

RULE 10: I WILL BE SAFE
ಹಿ

Learn to protect yourself by seeing to it that your health care professionals maintain common safety procedures. Before anyone touches an open wound or dressing, be sure they wash their hands. You learned this basic rule of hygiene as a child, yet sometimes even physicians forget when they are hurried. Insist on it. You can pick up viruses and infections in a hospital. Cancer patients have to be especially careful about these things. If a nurse or other health care worker has a cold, say, "I'd feel more comfortable if you wore a mask when you are taking care of me — at least until you're rid of that cold."

Along the same lines, always make sure that the needle puncturing your vein is new and clean. One-time disposable needles should be used. If you are unsure, ask that the needle be unwrapped in your presence.

Be careful about unnecessary exposure to radiation. If a patient in your room is about to be X-rayed, ask the technician to wait until you can leave the room and the process is completed. You don't need a gratuitous dose of radiation. If you are immobilized, insist on the protection of an insulated apron. I did this once, to the extreme annoyance of the technician, who had to go back to the Radiology Department to get an apron for me.

* * * * *

Don't be afraid to complain if you feel you're getting overexposed to the X-ray machine. I was once subjected to several retakes of a mammogram by an inexperienced student technician. Who knows how much longer I'd have been there if I hadn't demanded that the radiologist take over.

Speak up if you ever feel you are in jeopardy. You are already ill; you don't need any other harm done to you.

As you institute your patient's rights, bear in mind your obligations as a patient, to your physician, his staff, to the hospital and the health care professionals. Respect their schedules and routines as well. You're entitled to have your needs met, but only if they're appropriate. Further, you're entitled to have them met in a reasonable amount of time — but appreciate that, like you, physicians and hospital staff have their priorities.

On behalf of all cancer patients, I offer a plea to all

medical personnel. Let patients know that you hear them. You may have no idea what a comfort it is merely to have their pain acknowledged. It makes a difference to feel the touch of a sympathetic hand, to get a lumpy pillow fluffed, to hear the words, "I'm here; you're not alone," or "It's rough," or "It's scary." Anything that tells a patient, "We know you're hurting and we care," means more than you could imagine.

PART III

THE TREATMENT-GAME PLAN

Chapter 11

THE SURGICAL EXPERIENCE:
WHAT TO ASK (AND DO)
BEFORE THEY CUT

The typical first response to the shock of a cancer diagnosis is to throw yourself into whatever the doctor suggests, and be carried along like a leaf in a storm-swollen stream.

Over and over again in counseling cancer patients and their families, I hear, "But the doctor has already scheduled surgery." My answer to that is: "So what?" Schedules can be changed; decisions can be revoked. This is your life. Are you going to worry about hurting the doctor's feelings? Whatever you decide, your doctor will survive. But you have to ask yourself: Will I survive?

UNDERSTANDING SURGERY

ટ✵

With surgery, you literally put your life in someone else's hands, so it is important that you and your surgeon understand each other. Your surgeon should know what you want. Your doctor can't respect your wishes if he or she doesn't know what they are. The physician may have to make decisions about your body while you are undergoing an operation; by making your best hopes clear, you can assure that those decisions aren't arbitrary.

Often a doctor schedules a patient for surgery within days of the initial diagnosis. Surgery is still one of the most effective means of treating some types of cancer, but it's important for you to determine if it is the best alternative in your case.

When the doctor determines that surgery is called for, be sure that the treatment plan is explained to you fully and clearly. This information is your right. It's very important for you to understand. Ask what results the doctor expects. Are there side effects? How long will healing take? Are there any alternatives? If the surgery is exploratory, are there other means of reaching the same conclusion? Ask if sophisticated diagnostic equipment might render exploratory surgery unnecessary. This is also the time to ask about chemosensitivity assay testing or other tests mentioned in Chapter 6. If this is too daunting for you, enlist your family physician, a relative or close friend to do it for you, but make sure it is done.

In *Beyond the Relaxation Response*, cardiologist Dr. Herbert Benson counsels that patients whose doctors suggest surgery should be sure it's right for them. "Doctors are too quick to choose the surgical option when it isn't really necessary," he writes. Benson proposes that patients seek doctors who are very precise about surgical follow-up (so that no additional damage is done).

Surround yourself with expertise, but don't be swept away by jargon — if you hear medicalese and don't understand it, get it cleared up before you make any decisions.

UNDERSTANDING PATHOLOGY

The specific expertise of a pathologist (a medical doctor trained to interpret and diagnose changes in body tissues caused by disease) is crucial. If you require surgery, the pathologist often will direct its course. This doctor ultimately decides whether your tumor is benign or malignant. I say *decides* because that determination is not always so easy to make.

A friend who worked at the National Cancer Institute told me, "You'd be amazed at the number of experts — these are the top pathologists in the country, possibly in the world — who disagree, at times, on whether a cell is cancerous or not."

At your request, your slides or tissue samples can be shipped to the cancer center, hospital or laboratory of your choice. In one year, pathologists at the Sylvester CCC University at Miami Medical School examined 5.5 million slides.

Pathology departments at other Comprehensive Cancer Centers also work with a tremendous volume of materials sent for their analysis. I would feel comfortable with a pathology report from any of them. Just ask your doctor to send your slides to a cancer center for a second interpretation. However the doctor reacts, don't get defensive; this is not an unusual request.

UNDERSTANDING ANESTHESIA

The physician we hear very little about is the anesthesiologist. He is a crucial member of your surgical team. During surgery, he is as essential to a successful outcome as your surgeon. Yet we often meet him only the night before surgery, if at all. Some of the questions you might want to ask your anesthesiologist beforehand are:

* Is he certified by the American Board of Anesthesiology?
* Is he the one who will administer the anesthesia?
* Does he have a team that he works with?
* Could you be getting somebody else?
* If it is somebody else, will he also be board certified?

Ask about general versus local anesthesia. If you have a choice, local may be the safer way to go. During general anesthesia, the anesthesiologist puts you to sleep with any of an assortment of drugs. He then inserts a tube through your mouth into your windpipe and controls your breathing by regulating the ventilator to which the tube in your windpipe is attached. In addition to this crucial role, he must observe closely and regulate your blood pressure, blood oxygen, body temperature, brain activity and other vital signs. Small wonder that I urge you to be sure he is qualified and board certified.

The local or regional techniques block sensations to a *specific* area of the body and are certainly preferable because patients aren't exposed to possible dangerous ramifications of general anesthesia.

If your condition requires that you be scheduled for many hours of surgery, a regional block eliminates the need to be under a general anesthesia for so long a period of time. For patients with a specific allergy or heart or lung problems, local anesthesia may be their only option. It would be wise to ask your anesthesiologist, "Can my surgery or this procedure be performed with local or regional anesthesia?" If the answer is "Yes," I wouldn't personally consider going any other way.

The field of anesthesiology has changed considerably in recent years. Sophisticated innovations such as the pulse oximeter and a carbon dioxide monitor reduce the risk in general anesthesia. These new devices (and others that have been developed), allow for much more safety and less undesirable side effects, and postoperative complications, so be sure to discuss this with your anesthesiologist.

If you have had extensive bridgework, as I have, you should be sure to bring it to the attention of your anesthesiologist, especially if he will be inserting tubes into your throat to facilitate breathing. This will alert the anesthesiologist to be very careful while inserting any tubes into your throat so no damage will be done to your bridgework. You can end up with costly and uncomfortable damage if he's not.

PREPARING FOR SURGERY

Before a scheduled surgery, most hospitals ask the patient to come in beforehand for pre-admission. At that time, your insurance information and medical history are taken, routine blood and urine tests are done, a chest X-ray, cardiogram, or whatever else has been ordered will be performed. When you make this appointment, do ask if you can have a pre-admission anesthesiology consultation at the same time. Many hospitals offer this option. You'll be asked about many things like any medications you use, allergies, smoking, alcohol habits, any reactions you or family members have had to anesthesia, and others items which are all factors that can affect your reaction to the anesthesia. Be sure to tell all.

When surgery (or any other treatment) is prescribed and you are seeking a second opinion, it also is important to get a second reading of X-rays, scans, mammograms (X-rays of the breast), and other diagnostic information. A doctor's reading of test results is usually a matter of interpretation. In deciphering this raw data, the physician must bring an entire career of experience and expertise into play. What one doctor disregards may set off warning bells in another.

If a doctor makes you uneasy, he or she may not be the physician for you. If his exam is haphazard, it may be a small thing, but it can tell you a lot about the doctor.

Ask your doctor what you can expect when you wake up after surgery. You may need special care. If he thinks this is likely, ask if you should engage private nurses or ask a family member or a friend to help if you can't afford nurses for the first day or two. Usually, regular nurses are more than helpful and can do a lot of good for you, but sometimes you need the extra personal attention that overburdened staff nurses can't supply.

Faced with something as scary as surgery, I always find it reassuring to have a nurse close by, someone whose hand I can squeeze. If a family member can stay with you during the postoperative period, so much the better. But all this should be worked out with your doctor well in advance.

Sometimes, if close postoperative monitoring is needed, patients are taken directly from the operating room to an intensive care unit. If that's a possibility in your case, you want to know ahead of time. Waking up in intensive care when you don't expect to is scary. You open your eyes and see a lot of nurses working intensely on their patients. You see other patients hooked up to heart monitors, intravenous tubes, respirators and lots of mysterious gear. You notice that the nurses don't make idle conversation; the unit is quiet and a sense of urgency fills the air. With dawning consciousness, you realize that you, too, are attached to sophisticated equipment. If this comes as a surprise, you may think, Oh, dear, this is it. I'm going to die, and similar dire thoughts that may have no relationship to reality at all.

Slow down. Be prepared. Talk to your surgeon in advance to prevent this kind of stress, which is the last thing you need. Ask about the possibility of being in intensive care, of being on a monitor, of getting blood transfusions or needing oxygen. The more you are prepared psychologically, the better it will be. Studies have shown that those patients who had a positive attitude before facing surgery had better outcomes.

Most patients need to have things explained to them in detail. They need to know the reasons why things are being done. When they're ignored, or given no explanations, they might think the worst. In this weakened state, they may find that they say negative things to themselves. They worry if the doctor isn't telling them anything, if he's not coming around, things must be pretty bad. When they are well-informed and well-prepared, most patients will find it much easier to think positively.

Advance preparations pave the way to peace-of-mind. Alert your surgeon to your personal strengths and weaknesses. Explain what you need in terms of emotional support and what kinds of things will help you physically. Make yourself understood so that your doctor is armed with the knowledge needed to ensure that your postoperative hospital time is a positive, healing experience.

. . . PERSONAL PERSPECTIVE
ဗ

I once dealt with a surgeon who was to remove two small lumps on my back. Because there was a possibility that it could have been a recurrence of a malignancy of the lymph system, I was petrified. I had, of course, checked with my oncologist who assured me that a good general surgeon was qualified to remove the lumps. But there was another consideration. If the pathology report on the lumps showed malignancy, the oncologist wanted the tissue to be preserved in a special way and sent to him for further examination. He asked that my surgeon contact him so that he could discuss the tissue preservation medium that should be used.

The surgeon had assured me that he would call my oncologist up north for instructions on this point. The day my surgery was scheduled, I went to the doctor's office, and the nurse put me in the surgical room. She asked me to sign a consent form. When I saw that the form was not filled out, I told her that I couldn't sign it.

"Oh, the doctor will fill it in later," she said.

I would no sooner sign a blank consent form than pay a bill with a blank, signed check. I replied, "Then I'll fill in the particulars before I sign this."

I wrote in that two lumps side by side were to be removed from my left lower back and added that the tissue was to be preserved according to instructions from my oncologist and sent to him. The nurse read it and said, "We can't preserve tissue that way in the office. That would have to be done in the hospital."

I was floored. "Why wasn't I told this in the first place?" I asked. "Why did the doctor have me come to the office if he knew that what I requested couldn't be done here?"

The nurse had no answer and walked out, obviously exasperated. She returned with the doctor. He stood in the hall outside the room and addressed me in a very loud, authoritative voice, which I was sure my husband could hear way out in the waiting room. "There's really no need for the tissue to be sent to your oncologist. I'm sure the lump is benign."

"But did he say it wasn't necessary?"

He did not, the surgeon told me, and admitted upon further questioning that he hadn't talked to my oncologist. He hadn't bothered to call.

When I insisted on abiding by my oncologist's recom-

mendations, the surgeon assured me that he had done a year of pathology and was well qualified to know whether the lump was malignant or benign.

"That's not the point," I said. "If it turns out to be malignant, my oncologist wants the tissue for further study."

The surgeon snapped at me, "Well, if you insist on being part of their study, maybe you ought to go up north for this."

I was devastated by his aggressive, intimidating manner. I turned away from him and the officious nurse and tried to collect myself. Tears welled in my eyes. I was frightened and humiliated. I felt like a non-person. I was ready to go home in defeat. But, I told myself not to do that. This was exactly why I was telling people to stand up for themselves. I had to get a handle on myself—and speak up!

I took a deep breath and said, "You've got to be kidding. You're not telling me to get on a plane and go all that way to have two little lumps removed. I assure you, I couldn't care less about their studies. What I want is the best possible care for myself. I'll be guided by what my oncologist says."

The surgeon grudgingly agreed to try to reach my oncologist. I dashed out to the waiting room to tell my husband what had happened (it's important to have someone to back you up at times like this). I told Seymore that if the surgeon couldn't reach my oncologist, I'd tell him that my husband insisted that the procedure be done in the hospital.

As it turned out, the surgeon reached my oncologist, who still wanted the tissue — if malignant — preserved as per instructions and shipped to him. The surgeon had no choice. My procedure was done the next day — in the hospital.

Chapter 12

THE RADIATION EXPERIENCE:
A PRACTICAL GUIDE

Radiation treatment goes by many names. It is also known as cobalt treatment, irradiation, radiation therapy, radiotherapy, X-ray therapy, and X-ray treatment. It consists of using X-rays at high levels — tens of thousands of times the amount used in a chest X-ray — to destroy the ability of cells to grow and divide. While it affects both normal and diseased cells, most normal cells are able to recover quickly.

Radiation can cure. Radiation can alleviate pain. And radiation can kill. The risks involved in radiation therapy are widely known. It's no wonder that cancer patients usually approach it with reluctance and fear. It can be a very scary experience.

UNDERSTANDING RADIATION

It may be useful to you to understand that a *radiologist* is a medical doctor whose speciality is to read X-rays and scans and furnish interpretation and diagnosis. A *radiation oncologist or radiation therapist* (a physician who has a specialty in the use of radiation in the treatment of disease) prescribes and directs the course of radiation treatment.

Of the many variations of radiation therapy, *external beam radiation* (where the machine delivers the X-rays or gamma rays directly to the site of the tumor) is the standard type and is the most commonly used. *Internal radiation* is a procedure whereby radioactive material may be sealed in a container and inserted into a body cavity such as the uterus. Other methods of delivery can be by injection or by mouth.

Interstitial radiation or brachytherapy involves the insertion of needles into an organ such as a breast where a solid tumor exists. Tiny bits of radioactive material are implanted into the tumor through the needles that are placed in and around the tumor. These are usually left in place for several days after which they and the radioactive material with them are removed. A second type involves radioactive material which is permanently implanted directly into the affected organ and the radiation is released over a period of weeks or months.

Intraoperative radiation takes place in specially-designed operating rooms. As mentioned in Chapter 5, the operating rooms are equipped with radiation equipment to deliver radiation during surgery directly to the site of the patient's exposed tumor.

Ask your doctor if scarring and burning are avoidable. In my case, the radiation oncologist told me I could expect some burning around my neck where the radiation would be concentrated. He said it would look like a deep tan. So I was prepared for it in advance.

Ask your doctor how many patients he or she has treated with radiation for your condition and what the success rate was. If this is done with tact — not "How many of your patients lived, Doc?" but "In your experience, what is the success rate of this procedure? Does the cancer come back in some cases? How many?" If you are having radiation therapy after a lumpectomy for a breast cancer, ask if a mastectomy should be required at a later time, could the effects of the radiation prevent the surgery — you will be able to verify your doctor's experience without presenting a negative challenge.

As with all your doctors, develop a good rapport with your radiation oncologist. Communication is critically important. He must be alert to the signals of your body and your emotions.

Since radiation therapy doesn't usually warrant any substantial time out, maybe you can plan your own special treat, say for one weekend. It may be the theater, a ballgame, or a day out in nature and away from institutions. It may simply be to spend time with people you love. If you need a break, work on taking one. It will fortify you.

In terms of physical double-checking, cancer centers can fulfill informative roles in assessing radiation treatment. Yale University's Comprehensive Cancer Center often provides second opinions, and its Department of Therapeutic Radiology specializes in dosimetry, a state-of-the-art procedure for using complex computerized calculations to determine the exact dosages of radiation necessary in a particular case. Yale makes this service available to radiation therapists who can request a treatment plan determined by this sophisticated equipment. Yale also trains dosimetry specialists. The *dosimetrist* measures the exact dosage delivered with each treatment to ensure absolute accuracy in carrying out the radiation treatment protocol. Other Comprehensive Cancer Centers also use dosimetry.

When such detailed information is obtained routinely, you can be certain that you are in good hands. Even if you opt to undergo radiation therapy at a small community hospital and it doesn't employ a dosimetrist, it would be wise to ask your doctor to ask for a treatment plan to be calculated at a cancer center, or at least a second opinion from a qualified cancer center to verify the dose and treatment area that has been prescribed. You want to be sure because it may take up to three months to see the results of radiation therapy intended to be curative. Therapy for pain relief will work more quickly. In fact, the pain should decrease after a few treatments.

RESEARCHING NEW EQUIPMENT

A local newspaper reported an innovation in radiation therapy that the Radiation Department of Beth Israel

Hospital in New York City had developed. It was the use of a radiation cage to restrict the patient's movements, and thus reduce extraneous exposure to radiation during treatment. When you hear information like this on television or read it in the newspaper, never be afraid to tell your doctor, "I saw this on the news," or "I read an article about a new type of equipment. Would it be applicable in my case?" A competent doctor will not respond negatively to such questions. In the long run, your physician will value your awareness.

I followed up on the Beth Israel article and spoke to Dr. Bhadrasain Vikram, Director of the Radiation Department, who explained that this shell, as they called it, was custom-designed for each patient to keep the head more rigid during the delivery of the radiation. "This," he said, "would minimize the likelihood of unnecessary movement which could cause damage to healthy tissue." Dr. Vikram stressed that the experience of the radiation therapist might make the difference between success and failure.

An example of this is the linear accelerator, a very sophisticated piece of equipment that can be found in many small hospitals. A linear accelerator is a machine that accelerates electrons to high energies for the production of the X-radiations used in treatment. It is able to deliver exceedingly high doses of radiation to the area being treated. He pointed out: *But an important factor is the physicians who use the equipment and monitor the response and the reactions. It is similar to a general practitioner. He doesn't have the experience that an oncologist specializing in a specific type of cancer has.*

When I was researching treatment options for a client requiring head and neck surgery, I was referred to Dr. C. C. Wang at Massachusetts General Hospital, who, I was told, "is able to do radiation therapy in place of many surgeries."

He is Clinical Chief of the Department of Radiation Oncology at Massachusetts General and Professor of Radiation Therapy at Harvard Medical School as well as the author of *Radiation Therapy for Head and Neck Neoplasms: Indications, Techniques and Results*, Second Edition, published by Yearbook Publishers, Chicago, 1990.

Dr. Wang explained that certain cancers of the head and neck don't need surgery and that such tumors respond well to radiation therapy alone. In the case of advanced cancers, a combination of surgery and radiation is necessary, and the treatment is very complicated. He emphasized that the expertise of the physician in charge and the availability of treatment methods (if the hospital has the sophisticated equipment necessary) is crucial to a positive outcome. He uses a linear accelerator to deliver external beam radiation. A sophisticated delivery device is the intraoral cone, which shoots radiation directly into the tumor through the mouth without hurting the jaw. This allows the delivery of high-dose radiation to the tumor without doing damage to surrounding tissue.

In closing, Dr. Wang stressed again that patients should seek a second opinion from a radiation therapist who is an expert in that particular cancer treatment.

COPING WITH TREATMENT

Positive mind exercises are particularly important to radiation patients who may find it difficult to maintain a good attitude and not give in to fear and depression. It isn't easy, but it can be done.

Most people begin radiation treatment as in-patients. When an in-patient is brought to the radiation department for treatment, there's usually a backlog of other patients waiting to be treated. Some lie or sit quietly, locked into themselves. Others are very talkative, chatting about their cases and asking about yours. You see people who are desperately ill. It can be a weighty or a humbling ("there but for the grace of . . .") experience. My husband's brother had to have extensive radiation after lung surgery. He told me that sitting in the waiting room was worse than the treatment.

It's tough to keep your morale up in conditions like that. It is scary. But dwelling on the negative won't help you. You can switch off that scene and tune into your own positive thoughts. Not every patient is scarred or damaged by radiation. Most walk away from the treatments with minimal side effects. Tell yourself, "Radiation heals."

After a week or two as in-patients, most cancer patients come to the hospital for radiation treatments as out-patients. The tremendously difficult part for me, as for so many others, was transportation. One day, as an in-patient, you're being pushed along in a wheelchair by the transport crew. The next day, you're discharged and, as an out-patient, getting to the hospital is your own responsibility.

It isn't easy for an out-patient who has to depend on public transportation. It's so much easier to give up, missing treatments because you just don't feel up to it. But *get there*, no matter what.

Treatments that are not consecutive and consistent lose their efficacy. If you think you're too low physically or mentally to make it, pull yourself together. Your determination can make a difference in the outcome. Check to see if your hospital has a transportation van. Try the local chapter of the American Cancer Society. Ask your rabbi, minister or priest. Call a friend. Splurge on a taxi. But get your treatment every day.

Don't give up. Your most valuable asset as an out-patient is a positive, determined attitude. When your spirits start to sag, get help. Don't give in to depression and helplessness. Whatever you do, don't quit. The hospital can't help you unless you get yourself there. That's your job. Don't let anything defeat your resolve to get better.

You may spend much time alone in a situation that is particularly threatening. Get positive tapes working in your head: a doctor's hopeful remark, a parent's guidance, a favorite poem or prayer. Focus on the healing aspect of the treatment, even if you have to talk to the equipment. Tell it, "Okay, machine, do your job well. Go to work. Hit the spot. Knock it out. Get in there and make me well again. I want to live."

... PERSONAL PERSPECTIVE

When I received radiation therapy, I took it one day at a time. I made each day's treatment my goal for that day. Every morning when I woke up, nothing mattered but getting to the hospital at a specific time. I didn't project. If I'd ever let myself think about all the treatments to come, I'd have fallen apart. After I got my daily treatment, I would deal with the rest of the day.

On my way back to the hotel, if I could possibly manage it, I'd make it a point to stop somewhere for an hour or two along the way to shop or browse. Psychologically, it was vital to treat myself as if I was making it. Going straight back to the hotel room to go to bed after my treatment would have seemed like giving in. By pushing myself to do other things each day, I convinced myself that I was in control, that I wasn't really so sick. This was my action plan for survival.

In the evenings, my husband and I would go visiting. We had numerous friends and relatives in New York who were always happy to see us. Many a night, I could have done without it, but it was important to my husband. Seymore needs to be around people, especially in times of stress. I knew he was going through a lot. He never put pressure on me and I didn't want to be a drag. So, out we'd go.

I looked forward to week-ends. Every Friday, after I'd successfully pushed myself through another week of treatments, we'd take the subway out to Brooklyn to spend Sabbath with our friends. It was a wonderful source of strength and comfort.

Chapter 13

THE CHEMOTHERAPY EXPERIENCE :
YOU *CAN* HANDLE IT

Most people are aware of the existence of chemotherapy. Simply defined, it is no more or less than the *use of drugs to treat a disease*. We're told that it can cure some cancers, but not all; less often, are we told that many cancers would be hopeless without chemotherapy. We also read and hear about common side effects: hair loss, ulceration, loss of energy, pain, nausea, vomiting, diarrhea, constipation, increased vulnerability to infection, and more — an unpleasant gamut of physical reactions.

We are seldom reminded that not every patient has every side effect, and many people on maintenance doses of chemotherapy go to work and function normally.

The patients who come through chemotherapy most successfully are those who do not wallow in the doldrums of side effects. There is symptomatic relief available for almost every side effect except hair loss, and you can wear a wig until your hair grows back — which it will.

DEVELOPING A POSITIVE MINDSET

In most cases, if a patient develops a mindset — positive or negative — before chemotherapy, that mindset can direct the outcome and severity of side effects. This varies from person to person, of course, but a positive attitude is an asset during the course of treatment.

Patients who develop a positive outlook seem to tolerate chemotherapy better. Because of the very real connection between mind and body, I even wonder if chemotherapy might not be more effective for positive-minded individuals.

Try to identify something that will work for your good during chemotherapy. Visualize a healing medicine instead of something that will make you feel ill. See it as an ally that has been directed to destroy your tumor.

Some people find it easier to hear something in their imagination than to see something imaginary. If you are more auditory than visual, talk to yourself. Tell yourself — or tell the chemotherapy, "This is really working for me. Get in there and fight." You can even combine visualization and verbalization.

The *game plan* approach is one that can be used well with children receiving chemotherapy. The trick is to find the type of game or activity the child can relate to. An activity that might appeal to a child could be going out in a rowboat, with different members taking turns at rowing. One member could be responsible for the anchor, another for keeping the boat clean, someone to make sure the boat is seaworthy, and another to provide shelter when the boat is not in use. The child and the various medical professionals, parents and siblings can be seen as performing the different tasks of the crew members. Children can be given a hat, T-shirt or an article of clothing that could help them identify with the game or activity of their choice.

Build a set of *So whats?* about chemotherapy. "So what if it makes me throw up. That won't last forever. The medicine is working and that's what matters." In fact, vomiting — in association with many chemotherapies — usually lasts no more than a day. And for the nausea that lasts longer, modern medicine is constantly developing more and more effective antinausea medications. Tell yourself, "So what if I feel sick, things will return to normal, and I won't even remember this feeling." As with other traumas, tell yourself, "This too shall pass," or "So what if I lose my hair? It will grow back and it's a small price to pay when the purchase is my life." A way of making a minus into a plus is to say, "I guess a fringe benefit of losing my hair is I won't have to expend any energy to wash it and have to fuss with it," or "I'll save some money by not having to go to the beauty parlor or the barber."

Chemotherapy is not easy, but you don't have to dwell on it. You don't have to like it, but you don't have to crumble before it either.

GATHERING INFORMATION

ટ✿

The process of gathering all the information you need about chemotherapy is formidable. It is very difficult, sometimes impossible, to take in all this data and make an informed, unemotional decision by yourself. Instead of letting your emotions choke you, talk with someone else. Many volunteer programs can put you in touch with a person who has recovered from your type of cancer.

When the doctor recommends a protocol, ask questions. Find out if there are other treatment options. How long will this treatment take? Are there side effects? If you have a very large tumor, ask if it is in a place where radiation could be given to shrink the tumor, then followed with chemotherapy. Could that process improve your survival time? If there are other options, what should be considered in choosing this one form of treatment instead of another?

Ask about survival rates. How many patients is the figure based on? When I was researching one facility for a client, I was told that a particular clinical trial showed a 25-percent survival rate for his condition. I asked, "What is that statistic based upon? Does it mean one of four patients, five of 20, 25 of 100? And how long did they survive?" Keep asking, or, as mentioned, get someone — a friend or a professional — to ask for you.

A patient or caregiver who wants more extensive information about chemotherapy can read the book, *Choices:*

Realistic Alternatives in Cancer Treatment (Revised Edition) by Marion Morra and Eve Potts. It covers the whole gamut of cancer information, including chemotherapy. Nancy Bruning's pocket book, *Coping with Chemotherapy* is a good comprehensive guide to the special aspects of chemotherapy. Bear in mind, though, that both books are heavy and include medical material that not every cancer patient can handle.

DECISIONS, DISCUSSIONS AND DOSAGE
ह•

When Dr. Vincent T. DeVita, Jr., was Director of the NCI, he stressed the importance of high doses of chemotherapy. A May 8, 1986, article in *The Miami Herald* reported on Dr. DeVita's speech to 2,000 cancer researchers during the annual meeting of the American Association for Cancer Researchers. He said, "Thousands of cancer patients die needlessly each year because doctors lower chemotherapy doses."

He was further quoted as saying, "Well-meaning physicians have tended to lower chemotherapy doses because of unpleasant side effects for patients." Since many cancers will only respond to very aggressive chemotherapy, this may not be so well-meaning in the long run.

I spoke with specialists, some of whom are or were formerly at an NCI-sponsored cancer center, who advocate low-dose chemotherapy in overall doses equivalent to the high doses but are given over a calculated period of time different from the time schedule of a high-dose treatment plan. This is different from those physicians who simply lower the total recommended dose of chemotherapy. I was told by proponents of lower doses over a longer period of time there is no difference in the overall outcome. Both approaches work equally as well.

I have worked with many patients whose cancer had metastasized who expressed their anger at not having been given high-dose chemotherapy in the beginning. Many believe their cancers would not have spread if they had the high doses or that *big blast* up front.

If this is an important factor for you, you need to ask your oncologist if either low-dose or high-dose chemotherapy is an option in your case. If it is and you are given all the information about each type of treatment, you can make the best decision for which approach you can live with, both emotionally and physically. The odds are that if you are an aggressive patient, you are more likely to opt for the high dose, and if you are a more passive patient, you will probably go for the lower dose over a longer period of time.

However, if you are in a situation where you have to continue working or have small children or grandchildren and you want to feel as well as possible in order to care for or be with them, the low-dose approach with the milder side effects might be the way to go. This may be less debilitating and allow you more freedom physically. These aspects with regard to treatment need to be explored with your oncologist and/or a counselor.

This is the time when the prognostic tests you read about in Chapter 6 that can indicate a tumor's potential to spread ought to be discussed. Given all the pros and cons on their accuracy and reliability, I have found that most patients can handle being involved in discussing the results of these tests and how much they want the results to influence their choice of treatment. When given all the facts and allowed to be an active participant in the decision-making, you can be more confident about the treatment and thus handle it in a more positive manner.

COPING WITH SIDE EFFECTS
(THEY'RE ONLY TEMPORARY)

When faced with side effects of chemotherapy, such as hair loss, most women do what I did at first: go to a department store and buy a wig out of a box. An option I found more satisfying was to go to a wig salon that deals exclusively in selling wigs and cutting and styling them to suit your face and to look more natural. Go to a salon before chemotherapy, before you lose your hair, so that the stylist can help you select a wig closest to your natural hair color and style. You can wear your hair as you always have, or you can take the opportunity to make a change.

If you don't have medical insurance to cover the expense and you can't afford a wig, the American Cancer Society provides used ones at no charge. Call your local chapter. Wigs are also available for children. Some little girls may feel better about themselves wearing a natural-looking wig instead of a bandanna or scarf. Young boys may feel more comfortable with a hat or cap of their choice, such as a baseball cap from a favorite team. Men who don't relish the idea of being bald can always turn to a toupee.

Some chemotherapy patients can avoid hair loss by using an ice cap (also called a cold cap). Placed over your hair during chemotherapy infusions, this cap keeps your scalp very cold and prevents the chemotherapy from reaching your hair follicles, so your hair is less likely to fall out. The ice cap works for patients with certain cancers, but it is not indicated for patients with leukemia or lymphoma.

An ice cap is a great option, but make sure that the benefits outweigh the risks in your specific case. Only you can decide. If you face the possibility of hair loss, it'll help to be prepared and to keep reminding yourself the loss is temporary.

Nausea can be a real problem during chemotherapy as can ulceration of the mouth. Doctors can prescribe medication to help you through such side effects.

When I came back to Dana-Farber Cancer Institute in Boston for my first BACOD chemotherapy treatment, Dr. Skarin, my primary physician, was out of town, so Dr. Robert Mayer, mentioned in Chapter 10, started me off. Before the treatment, he gave me a shot of compazine for nausea and more compazine and sleeping pills to take when I arrived home (so I could sleep right through the postchemotherapy nausea). At that time, I was happy to get these goodies. Probably if I'd been more sophisticated then, I'd have panicked at the idea. What if I vomited in my sleep? I realize now that was why Dr. Mayer told Seymore to be sure somebody was with me during that period.

I slept away the day. The only thing I felt was a terrible frustration at the time wasted sleeping. Time had become very precious to me. But I am grateful that, through Dr. Mayer's ingenuity, I was spared the ordeal of ugly, painful retching. Years later, Dr. Mayer explained to me that his routine provided a structure, something he found cancer patients needed.

However, no one being treated with chemotherapy should take sleeping pills or any medication for that matter without first checking it out with their oncologist. There are many things available to blunt or mask nausea, and scientists continue to develop more effective antinausea agents.

Learn to look out for number one. Realize that most people you deal with regarding your illness have tunnel vision. Doctors, nurses, bookkeepers, and secretaries are all focused on what works best in the context of their own jobs. They don't always see the big picture from the patient's perspective. To survive physically, mentally and emotionally, you have to develop your own tunnel vision. You have to see only what is best for you. Whenever you can, in whatever way you can, you have to do everything in your power to protect yourself and make things easier for you.

Protect yourself during your chemotherapy. Make your needs clear. Conserve your energy. Cancer patients, especially young ones, have a tendency to run around a lot, as if proving to themselves that they're not really all that sick. Be with friends, keep involved, but pace yourself. No matter what your age, measure what you do in terms of maintaining enough resilience and strength to handle the treatment. Do what your body says you can handle, then stop.

Chemotherapy weakens your immune system, lowering your ability to fight infection. When you get your treatments, keep out of crowds as much as possible. If someone near you in a group or even on a plane starts coughing or sneezing, keep your distance. Discreetly turn your face away and hold a tissue over it, as if you need to blow your nose.

Make it a point to carry a sweater or jacket with you

at all times, even in hot weather. You have to watch out for extremes of air-conditioning. Carry an umbrella to avoid getting drenched in sudden, unexpected downpours. During a rainy season, it's easy to pick up a cold or infection. That's a normal nuisance for most people, but it can be a disaster for a cancer patient.

While you're on chemotherapy, keep in touch with your body. Report any significant change to your physician. It may be a warning signal or side effect of the treatment. For example, overpowering weakness may be a sign of anemia.

Being on chemotherapy is at times like being on a roller coaster. You may hear your counts are up, your counts are down, you're in remission, we've found a new spot. One week you may be feeling great and able to get around. Then suddenly you crash. Blood counts go down a week to ten days after the infusion. Not every doctor remembers to tell this to his patients. If the count is very low, you can feel so weak you may think you are going to die. When this happened to me, I made myself remember the times I had snapped out of that feeling and made a come back. Many patients need repeated blood transfusions; that doesn't mean they are not going to make it. It's important if you are experiencing the down-side of chemotherapy to remind yourself that things can pick up again. Keep your sights on the up-side when you find yourself on that roller coaster.

Watch your weight. Many chemotherapy protocols are tied to body weight. After you lose a certain amount of weight, the chemical dosage that your body can tolerate decreases. Your dose needs to be adjusted accordingly.

Most physicians routinely have their patients weighed before each infusion. Ask if your chemotherapy is calculated according to your weight. If so, keep your own records of your weight and of how many grams of chemotherapy you are getting. Learn how much weight loss you can sustain before your dose needs to be reduced. If you sustain a considerable weight loss, bring it to the attention of your physician before your infusion. Slip-ups can take place in busy offices or hospitals. It happened to me once.

Coping with chemotherapy is not easy. I went through terrible agonies. But they are over. And if I had to do it again, I'd opt for the same thing. Without aggressive chemotherapy and the high doses of methotrexate, I might not have survived.

Chemotherapy has been responsible for countless remissions and cures where other treatment plans failed. Hang in there. Remember your priorities; keep your mind fixed on a good outcome.

. . . PERSONAL PERSPECTIVE

My introduction to chemotherapy came when my physician diagnosed the non-stop, severe back pain I felt as a blockage of the kidney caused by enlarged lymph nodes. The lymphoma was back. The physician recommended that I start on BACOD (five chemotherapies: Bleomycin, Adriamycin, Cytoxin, Oncovin and Decadron), an aggressive combination of chemotherapy drugs. Dana-Farber added high-dose methotrexate. I was given an information sheet about methotrexate. More scary news. I would have to drink quarts of water. Every time I urinated, I would have to check the pH (acidity) of my urine. If it went over or under the acceptable limits, I was to call the emergency number at the adult clinic immediately for instructions.

My other nemesis was the leucovorin rescue, which protects a patient from some of the harmful effects of high doses of the methotrexate. I had to take a prescribed number of pills every four hours. I needed to have a blood test at the center, and I would call in for them to tell me whether I had to increase or decrease the pills. And I didn't feel well at all during that period.

In the infusion room at Dana-Farber, I had my choice of several chairs, recliners or beds. Everything was arranged to help the patient be as comfortable as possible.

As I settled in for my first methotrexate treatment, I kept working on the internal mindset that I wasn't going to get nauseous. I wasn't going to lose control and vomit. I would handle it. Remembering how I coped with morning sickness when I was pregnant, I brought soda crackers along. I asked the nurse for ginger ale and for cracked ice to chew. I stirred a little sugar into the ginger ale to get the gas out as my mother used to do for me when I was sick. I was determined these things would work. And they did!

Not long into the methotrexate infusion, my eyebrows and forehead began to itch. I put my hand to my forehead and felt a few welts. Pretty soon, the itching spread. I started to panic. I called the nurse. She looked closely at my face, stopped the IV immediately and quickly paged Dr. Arthur Skarin, my primary physician.

He showed up in minutes and administered an antihistamine to ward off an allergic attack, slowed the rate of infusion and instructed the nurse to stick to me like glue. One or two new welts appeared, but the nurse monitored me closely, and the doctor kept coming back to check. I was terrified, but it was reassuring to know that Dr. Skarin would be right there if anything happened. I was able to take the whole dose.

A month passed and Dr. Skarin examined me closely before my second BACOD chemotherapy treatment. He poked around my spleen area, and suddenly his face lit up. He looked at me with that smile of his and said, "Gee, this is great! I can almost feel right through to your back!" I had received very aggressive chemotherapy, a BIG blast. Thank goodness, it did the job. I had responded tremendously to the chemotherapy. My spleen had gone down to its normal size.

I kept my positive mental tapes spinning, and I got through the more than ten months of heavy-duty treatment. I have very little memory of the suffering I endured. My attitude now is, "So I had to go through pain. It was worth it. Life is beautiful. I thank God every day that I'm here to enjoy it."

PART IV

IN LIMBO

Chapter 14

RECURRENCE — HERE WE GO AGAIN:
SIGNS, FEARS, FACTS AND SOLUTIONS
THE SECOND TIME AROUND

Many cancer patients emerge victorious over their cancer and never have to confront it again, but some — like me — face a recurrence of the disease. It isn't any better the second time around, but at least you know you can bear it, and with help even beat it, because you already have.

LEARNING ABOUT
RECURRENCE

If you are undergoing after-care, find out from your doctor exactly what kind of recovery record your cancer has. If you lack any knowledge about the kind of cancer you had, learn it now. Know your enemy. Often, well-meaning family members may shield you from the whole picture. Ask, "Is this a recurring type of cancer? Is it particularly aggressive or rare?" Don't shy away from knowing about your disease. You need this information to keep on top of your case.

Be sure to ask if there are any tests that specifically identify recurrence of your type of cancer. With new advances, tests and treatments change constantly, so keep checking with your oncologist. You may be a candidate for one of these tests, or your physician may know of others. Remember, the tests that identify early recurrence or metastasis are described in Chapter 6. Check with qualified laboratories that are up-to-date on the latest prognostic tests.

Inquire if your physician thinks you are a candidate for any preventative care, such as chemotherapy.

LISTENING TO
YOUR BODY

The scariest part about cancer the second time around is that you already know how swiftly and totally this insidious enemy strikes, how brutally it devastates your body. Cancer patients are fearful of the slightest indication that something may be amiss, but denial and avoidance are not the wise approach. Act at the earliest signal of any trouble.

In defense of doctors, many patients are extremely sensitive and do rush to their physicians with even the slightest problems. Doctors can keep this in perspective and still be compassionate. The complaints cancer patients have, such as weakness, pain or bowel irregularities, may be the lingering effects of treatments and not symptoms of disease. But patients need to be assured, and reassured, that their symptoms are normal and that the doctor knows there's always the chance that something more serious may be happening.

Cancer is a sneaky, cagey enemy. Sometimes the best doctors and the most sophisticated equipment fail to detect its presence.

In fact, the December, 1988, issue of *American Health* carried a story, "When The Patient Knows Best" by Dr. Stephen A. Hoffman, a Harvard Medical School internist. Dr. Hoffman writes of a case where his patient was more reliable than the lab results of the patient's blood test. Dr. Hoffman cautions, "Normal tests don't necessarily add up to a normal person." In many cases, the patient's account matters more to him than sophisticated diagnostic tests, electrocardiograms or X-rays. Hoffman tells his patients,

"Your doctor needs your account of how you feel."

Total faith and dependence on one doctor is not unusual. It is integral to the doctor-patient relationship, although it has obvious risks. Doctors have to recognize both the intrinsic nature of this bond and the power it invests in them.

Effective care requires teamwork between doctor and patient. Be watchful. Share your observations, fears or suspicions with your teammate.

You are the expert on your body; the physician is the expert on treatment. You must supply the facts, but the doctor must interpret them and follow through.

As Dr. Stephen Hoffman said: "We doctors need to remember that not everything important can be measured and what can be measured may not be important. When push comes to shove, it's often the person who should have the last word."

. . . PERSONAL PERSPECTIVE

ৡৡ

Only through my own persistence I discovered that my cancer was a recurring type. The many doctors I had seen failed to tell me this. I found this out a year after my radiation treatments.

I was devastated, but I handled this news. What was almost unbearable was that of all the physicians I saw during my follow-up care up to that time, not one explained I had a recurring type of lymphoma; nor did they instruct me as to what symptoms to look for.

I felt betrayed by the doctors for not letting me know all the aspects of my condition. It was important for me to know. Many patients have complained they were not told all the particulars of their diseases. When the disease recurred, they felt tremendous anger at their physicians who hadn't kept them fully informed.

I was in follow-up care 18 months before the recurrence was diagnosed. I saw seven doctors during that time. I persisted in telling them I continued to feel weak and described my symptoms. They found nothing. My last oncologist, the late Dr. Jacob Colsky, listened intently to my complaints: the pain in my throat which felt like I had a lump there. I described an attack of excruciating kidney-like pains I had about ten months prior to my visit, yet the X-ray films of my kidneys showed nothing, and how my previous oncologist never pursued it further.

Dr. Colsky explained that sometimes lymphomas recur. "The pain you had," he told me, "could have been blockage of the kidney caused by enlarged malignant lymph nodes in your stomach." He asked me to sign a release for my hospital records. He wanted his pathologist to look at my slides and he wanted me to have a gallium scan. "They are 85 percent accurate for picking up signs of a lymphoma," he said. My gallium scan was negative. He asked me to come back in a month. He wanted to stay on top of my case. At last I knew I was in the care of a competent, cautious physician I could trust.

One morning, after a night of non-stop pain, I called and insisted on speaking to Dr. Colsky. He saw me right away, and I learned my lymphoma was back.

My persistence in finding a doctor who listened to me, who tested out his and my suspicions of recurrence, paid off. I was right to follow my instincts that something was wrong, but it was devastating to have to face a fresh bout with that treacherous disease.

I don't think all those doctors who examined me overlooked some obvious signal. There wasn't anything to see; but I knew something was wrong. I could feel it. My body told me so. Further tests might have identified it. Sometimes you know best.

Chapter 15

Remission! Home At Last:
STAYING ON TOP OF THE FACTS

Remission means a miracle has happened. The cancer is gone, completely or partially. With complete remission, all symptoms and clinical signs of cancer have disappeared, though cells may remain in the body. For many cancers, a five-year remission is considered a cure. In partial remission, some of the clinical signs and symptoms are gone, but not all. Either type of remission can last weeks or years.

The media are full of grim statistics about dying, about how the odds for surviving the worst kinds of cancer aren't getting any better. But they don't say that some people have survived even the most hopeless forms of cancer. There are survivors of lung cancer. There are survivors of liver cancer. Pancreatic cancer is said to be one of the very worst varieties, and yet within my own limited circle of cancer patients, I know at least two people who have survived it.

Lots of people survive cancer. Lots of people who have cancer lead active, productive, fulfilling lives. People need to hear this message.

Often those who have had cancer find their personal good news difficult to accept. We want and need remission so badly that when it comes we're afraid to believe it. We're apprehensive that, as in the movies, the moment we think the monster is really gone it will come back meaner than ever. We're in limbo.

Inevitably you run into people, including doctors and nurses, who ask, "How long have you been in remission?" If you're lucky enough to be able to answer two or three years, or more, they beam at you and say, "So, you're cured! That's great!"

I usually answer, "I hope so, please God." But inside I cringe. It seems like tempting fate.

Most of the cancer survivors I've worked with feel the same way. On the other hand, we also need and appreciate encouragement. We're trying to think positively and get on with our lives, but cancer patients in remission feel like they're living with a sentence over their heads. Fear lurks just below the surface —fear of recurrence, fear that a new cancer could suddenly break out in a fresh location. So we don't like to hear, "You're okay now!" A cautious, "You must feel very special," or "That must have been some ordeal you went through. Let's hope your good news continues," or "I'm so happy for you," is much easier to take.

USING YOUR FEAR
OF RECURRENCE
ह৺

Our fears are not unfounded. A sizable body of research indicates that after ten or more years some treatments can cause new cancers to develop. It creates a lingering impression, but that's not a reason to give into fear. I know I must not.

A classic study revealed that university students who smoke heavily are the most reluctant to see a doctor when they have a deep cough or breathing difficulties — anything that could be related to their smoking habits. Fear makes them procrastinate. Patients in remission must not give in to this kind of apprehension. Fear intensifies pain. The gnawing anxiety that this new ache or pain might be cancer makes it much harder to endure. Your splitting headache is probably a reaction to tension, but what if it lasts two weeks? Is it worth being anxious when a visit to your doctor could put your mind at ease?

When I'm apprehensive, I overreact. Every twinge portends disaster. Some people have the opposite reaction: complete denial. They ignore even severe pain that should be checked. Be watchful. When something isn't right, discuss it with your doctor, but try not to let either fear or denial endanger you.

REMAINING VIGILANT

Remission means follow-up, continuing care and watchfulness. This is a special time. No longer are you fighting against the tide. Your treatment course, whatever it may have been, has delivered you into calmer waters. You have fought the insidious invader and, at this moment, you have the upper hand. You are on top of your case, and you want to stay on top.

Patients in remission can do a lot to minimize the risks of recurrence. Nobody knows what causes cancer — not the whole picture, anyway. But we do know that certain people have a propensity for it. If you've had cancer, your body may have that propensity. Be especially watchful. My medical history tells me that I am such a person, so I'm very careful. If there is something in my life that may be cancer-causing, I weed it out.

You have learned the truth of "an ounce of prevention is worth a pound of cure." Be sure your doctor is prevention-oriented and then form a partnership to hunt down problems before they have a chance to grow.

Be diligent for yourself. Even your oncologist can sometimes fail to recommend all the tests you need to detect any new cancer. Let's look at some of the cancer-related testing you should pursue, and then we'll discuss the follow-up care you need in terms of your general health. It is usual for follow-up care to include routine blood tests, chest X-rays and either mammograms or prostate exams. Other tests might depend on your type of cancer.

Every cancer is different and the direct follow-up care for each is different. So, be sure you have a competent cancer specialist on your team.

During follow-up, your oncologist may suppose you are also seeing an internist and other specialists. If you are not, you should be. Your internist can track many aspects of your health that don't fall into your oncologist's purview.

It is important to stay on top of other routine check ups, including seeing your eye doctor and dentist. Many people who have had radiation to the head or neck need extra fluoride treatments for their teeth. Watch out for unnecessary exposure to radiation from those dentists who routinely take X-rays every six months. You don't need the excess radiation; speak up and look out for your own safety.

Remember that cancer care comes in addition to your usual health maintenance routine, not instead of it. Follow-up is also the time to ask your doctor about adding vitamins A, C, E, and selenium to your usual health care routine (see Chapter 18). If your physician can't advise you on nutrition, consult a nutritionist or qualified health counselor. You might want to visit a doctor who specializes in preventive medicine. These practitioners have had extensive education in nutrition, vitamin, mineral and other supportive therapy in order to build up and maintain the immune system.

Do all you can for your general health in terms of wise nutrition, moderate exercise and avoidance of stress and bad habits. The hope is that you will have a long, strong life with no cancer recurrence. But if there is a recurrence, you'll be better equipped to fight it if you've taken care of yourself.

You can develop an early warning system attuned to what is going on in your body. I rely on body signals for clues to my physical condition. If I suddenly catch colds easily or get infections that heal slowly, I check myself out. "Okay, Sarah, what's the problem?" Maybe you're running around too much, not getting enough rest, or under too much stress.

MINIMIZING STRESS
ह़✿

Your body is your best follow-up monitor. If you are
feeling stress, anxiety or fatigue, your body is letting you
know that your immune system isn't up to par. You want to
maintain the strongest, healthiest immune system you can as
your first, best line of defense against a cancer recurrence.

The minute you realize that you're under stress, stop.
Hold everything. Stress can undermine your health. De-
fuse it before it hurts you. If you catch yourself in the
grocery store check-out line, seething with impatience
because the elderly person in front of you takes forever to
count his change, you're stressed out.

If you fret for hours before you sleep, if you nibble
junk food when you're not hungry, if you have started
biting your nails or snapping at your spouse, your children
or your parents, you are displaying signs of stress. You
need to talk to yourself, and the first thing to say is, "I'd
better calm down."

Ask yourself, "Am I going to let this get to me? Are
there things I can do to reduce my level of stress?"

Many times, you can't change a stressful situation
involving your family or friends or business. You may not
be able to remove yourself physically from stress-provok-
ing settings. But you can remove yourself emotionally. In
such cases, I consciously detach myself from whatever is
going on. I play my mental "So what?" and "Who says?"
tapes. "So what if you don't like what's happening?" "Who
says I have to have it my way?" Decide if the matter under
dispute is really important in the long run, and if it isn't,
step out of the flow of stress.

If you find that you're tired, rest. You can't do everything in one day. Define your limits and stick to them. So
what if the house is a mess? So what if the boss is in a rush?
Tomorrow is another day, and you have to be well before
you can accomplish anything.

Get your priorities straight. You've gone through a lot
with your body. Now it should be your top priority. Take
care of it. When I'm under stress and not feeling in top

form, I increase my vitamin C and vitamin B intake. I use
the relaxation therapies or techniques that helped when I
was in cancer treatment.

Don't be impatient. People recover at different speeds,
some quickly, some slowly. It can take a long time to feel
like your old self again.

. . . PERSONAL PERSPECTIVE
ও

*Like myself, many cancer patients and their families
from all parts of the world were at Rabbi Horowitz's New
England Chassidic Center, where they stayed while being
treated at the medical centers in Boston. I left the hospital
and went back to the Rabbi's home where I'd spent so many
weeks the previous summer at the start of my chemotherapy. Sitting around the kitchen table were Beryl with
his wife, their sick little daughter and their other children;
the couple from Haifa whose two-year-old son had a brain
tumor; the woman whose young child had Hodgkin's disease; Jason from Australia.*

*I looked at these brave people, at those beautiful,
desperately ill children, and I felt guilty. Who was I to gloat
over my good news in front of them? But I needed to tell them.
In a quiet voice, I said, "Thank God, everything is okay."*

*The room exploded with joy. They shouted, the women
hugged, the men grinned. I looked at Beryl. He positively
glowed. What a feeling I had witnessing these people laying
aside their own deep sorrows to revel in my good fortune!*

*Cancer patients and their families, those who never
had a brush with cancer, everyone wants to hear about
people making it — especially about those who, like myself,
had cancer in a very advanced stage. The families at the
Rabbi's center had seen me on days when I looked like I
wasn't going to survive, days when every step was a tremendous effort. For them to know that I had come through was
precious, hope-inspiring knowledge. If I could survive,
there was hope for their children, their spouses, themselves.*

*Although I am now in remission, I remain vigilant
and have many routine screening tests. Every two years I*

have a colonoscopy. Each year, I have a throat exam, thyroid function tests, a cardiogram, blood and urine tests, a chest X-ray, a mammogram, a pap smear and a gynecologic exam, and a general physical exam. Twice yearly, I have an eye exam, and I discuss with my oncologist whatever tests I hear of which may be useful and relevant.

During one eye exam, my opthalmologist told me that a spot on one pupil needed careful watching and should be rechecked in six months to see if it changed size since it could become melanoma. I was terrified about that spot, but my opthalmologist assured me that when such spots are found and are caught in time, surgery is generally curative.

Another physician told me I had symptoms of myasthenia gravis, which sometimes develops in people who have had lymphoma. I was scared enough to follow through on his recommendation that I have an electromyography, an extremely painful test. I tested negative, and an eminent neurologist in Boston diagnosed the condition as a form of muscular dystrophy.

As for the fact that any of these diseases might have dire outcomes, I don't dwell on it. I pray that they will come up with a treatment or cure which can benefit me. I awake each day and say, "Thank God I'm here!"

PART V

WHAT YOU CAN DO

Chapter 16

THE MIND-BODY CONNECTION:
DEVELOPING THE RIGHT ATTITUDE
FOR YOUR IMMUNE SYSTEM

What you feel emotionally and psychologically may change how your body fights disease. The latest scientific information strongly indicates that emotions affect the immune system. For a long time, many who counsel cancer patients have conjectured that the power to survive stems, in part, from the patient's own attitude and feelings, factors you can work on. Now science says that there is a mind-body connection.

CONFIRMING
THE CONNECTION

Psychoneuroimmunology (PNI), the field of medicine devoted to the study of the mind-body connection, has substantiated that your state of mind can activate some internal mechanisms that cause chemical reactions in your body, and these may be a factor in enhancing your immune system's effectiveness.

For example, experiments indicate that laughter apparently increases the activity level of the immune system, which sends out cancer fighting cells that attack tumors.

Positive emotions, such as love, faith and hope, appear to be physically good for you. PNI studies abound of how emotions affect the immune system. Actually, indications are that both the nervous system and the endocrine system affect the immune system, thus the immune system apparently is influenced by behavior. This may account for spontaneous remissions.

The study of the mind-body connection is not entirely new. The earliest medical practitioners were shamans, tribal *witch doctors* whose effectiveness, although limited, seems to have relied on their followers' belief in them.

There are many scientific landmarks in the study of the mind-body relationship, and a growing body of research indicates that personality may have a direct effect on surviving cancer.

Some of the researchers in our own century who contributed to the development of psychoneuroimmunology (PNI) were Doctors Franz Alexander; Hans Selye, organic chemist; Herbert Benson; Nicholas Cohen, immunologist; and Robert Ader, psychologist, who coined the phrase.

At Johns Hopkins University, a long-term study conducted by Caroline Bedell Thomas, M.D. and others, found that of nearly 1400 medical students given psychological tests in 1948, 48 had developed cancer by 1979. The questionnaires revealed that those who were ill tended to have a history of family turmoil. She found that subjects who were emotionally distant from one or both parents had a higher death rate from cancer.

In another long-term study, personality tests were administered to approximately 2000 male employees of Western Electric Company in Chicago. The results of a 20-year follow-up study were reported in 1987 by Richard Shekelle, Ph.D., and his colleagues and showed that those men who had been prone to depression were twice as likely to have died of cancer.

A study by Dr. Jimmie C. Holland, Chief of Psychiatry at New York's Memorial Sloan-Kettering Hospital, and other researchers found that depression, anxiety, confusion, tiredness and tenseness were more prevalent in pancreatic cancer patients than in patients with stomach cancer. The results of the study supported the belief of doctors treating cancer of the pancreas that patients were depressed and anxious before a diagnosis of pancreatic cancer was made.

A *Type C* (cancer-prone) personality was postulated by Lydia Temoshok, a psychologist at the University of California School of Medicine, as a result of her studies of patients at the Malignant Melanoma Clinic in San Francisco. She described a Type C person as one who has to feel in control, a domineering person unable to express emotion. Her research concludes that a Type C cancer patient might be expected to have a worse outcome than someone more emotionally expressive.

Psychologist and cellular biologist Joan Borysenko and her research group, mentioned in Chapter 2, demonstrated how certain chemicals (message carriers called neurotransmitters) in the central nervous system could affect an increase (or decrease) in immune system cancer-killing cells (T-cells). Their study confirmed the mind-body connection.

GROUP THERAPY
AND BREAST CANCER PATIENTS

PNI research has also led to the premise that one of the ways of increasing survival time may be to join a support group, an act that allows the patient a therapeutic vent for pent-up emotions.

Studies of women admitted to King's College Hospital in London for breast biopsies indicated that those who habitually suppressed anger showed a far greater incidence in malignancy.

A ten-year study of the effects of group therapy among women whose breast cancers had metastasized was published in the October 14, 1989, issue of the *Lancet*, a British medical journal. The study, conducted by David Spiegel, a psychiatrist at Stanford University and other researchers at both Stanford and the University of California at Berkeley, demonstrated that an experimental group of women in a therapy group survived 36 months whereas those in the control group who received chemotherapy alone without group support survived only 19 months.

In an article in the January, 1991, issue of *The Harvard Mental Health Letter*, Dr. Spiegel reported the women in the support groups in his study were helped to cope with the disease by learning to take charge of their lives, to be actively involved in their medical care, and to face their fears of dying.

The women were taught self-hypnosis to control pain and were encouraged to express their feelings, to deal with physical problems, and to be assertive with their physicians. The authors suggest that one of the factors which may have accounted for the prolonged survival among these women was the relief of depression facilitated by the group support. In the group setting, the women developed a sense of hope which led to improved appetite and the ability to follow through better with medical treatment.

In the same article, Dr. Spiegel expressed concern for patients who it was reported stopped their medical treatment and opted for a spiritualistic approach whereby they visualize their immune system killing cancer cells.

Dr. Jimmie C. Holland of Memorial Sloan-Kettering Hospital in the October 27, 1989, issue of *Science* found Spiegel's study scientifically sound although she voiced a fear that some alternative cancer therapists might use the results of the study to encourage cancer patients to abandon medical treatment. I have found this to be a significant problem in counseling cancer patients whereby many patients opting for positive-thinking alternative therapies were unwilling to consider medical treatment or investigational trials.

GAINING A
POSITIVE ATTITUDE
ॐ

The potential to be a survivor is your birthright; without it, you wouldn't have come this far on the perilous journey from helpless embryo to conscious adult. Though the mental baggage you acquire along the way may weaken or conceal it, the survival instinct never really leaves you. At any time in your life, you can learn to tap into its bottomless reserve.

Attitude is the key that unlocks the survivor within. Your desire to live has to be more than just a feeble hope. It has to be a consuming passion. Start by giving yourself an honest answer to a tough question: "Do I want to live?"

Sadly, the initial answer for some people is no. The pessimistic, defeated, already-ailing person may feel that life has lost meaning, that continuing on is too difficult. Existing psychological or personal relationship issues may be exacerbated by illness, leading to responses such as, "My family doesn't respect me; to them I am just the household slave." "Who cares about me?" "All they want me for is a paycheck." "What do I get out of life?" "I'm so alone. I don't really have a friend to my name. Why go on?"

If negative thoughts capture you, you'll see the cup as half empty. Although it takes only a minor shift of perception to see it as half full, most negative thinkers don't believe that change is possible.

One of the worst traits of pessimism is that it is self-renewing and self-fulfilling. Suppressed anger, fear or self-pity create an inability to think about anything but self. As a result, other people are perceived as being distant.

Perhaps loved ones can't reach across that space; perhaps relentless negative ideas block frightened, angry patients from really hearing anyone else. Either way, the feeling of worthlessness, the *poor me* attitude, is self-reinforcing.

The first step in making a transition from negative thinker to optimist is breaking out of the cycle of self-pity. A self-image is not how others see you, it is how *you* see yourself. No one else creates your self-image. Nothing anyone else says or does can change it unless you allow that change. If it needs changing, change it yourself.

Try not to get trapped inside your own head. Work on saying positive things about yourself to yourself. It's dangerous to play and replay internal tapes of powerlessness and unworthiness. If you're listening to tapes like that, give yourself a break. You deserve better.

When I get into that self-defeating cycle, it helps me to think about someone else. What can you do to make someone else's day brighter? Enjoy the difference your kind word or thoughtful action can make in another person's life. Let that lift your spirits and divert you from your own concerns.

Remember, your family and close friends also are having a hard time coping with your illness. They care about you. They are frightened for you. They don't want to be without you. They don't know how to act. Your pessimism can keep them at arm's length, even if they want to hold you and express their concern for you. *But they can only be a part of your life if you let them.*

Sharing yourself with others fills your own cup. The more we share with others, the closer we become. And without fail, the giver receives more than the receiver.

Weed out your negative attitudes. *Think positively* sounds like trite advice, but it works. Negative thinkers respond to the dread news that they have a malignancy with fateful resignation. Their listlessness, while masquerading as lack of interest in life, is really a failure to face up to emotions.

Reconnect with your feelings so you can harness fear and use it to fuel your counterattack. As I have said, cancer is a terrifying disease. It is something to cry about, but *don't wallow in your tears.* Get them out, and then get on with it! There is hard work to do.

Survival is, in some ways, a state of mind. No one, young or old, sick or healthy, knows when life will end. But no matter how long you survive — ten years, ten months or even ten days — if your attitude can be, "The cancer hasn't destroyed me yet. I'm in control. I'm living my own life and doing my own thing," then you are a survivor. You are living fully.

Your attitude makes all the difference. Your body is stimulated by motion. Joggers talk about the runner's high they experience, a kind of weightless, painless euphoria. Endorphins, secretions of the brain that produce a morphine-like effect and act as pain killers, were found to be secreted by runners during exercise. This may be why some people become addicted to running. Their addiction may be not to the running but to the euphoria they experience as a result of the secretion of endorphins. If this is the case, then exercise can be a double boost for cancer patients. They can benefit from the "high" feelings that are produced and these positive feelings can in turn have a beneficial effect upon the immune system.

It is interesting to note that morphine has a damaging effect on the immune system. Yet endorphins, which mimic morphine in their pain-relieving effect, conversely have a positive effect and enhance the production of T-cells, which fight infection. The "high" endorphins create could be a strong factor in this phenomenon.

Therapists now recognize how important it is to tap into this concept and get depressed patients moving. Your body is designed for movement. When it doesn't get it, you feel listless and depressed. Get a little exercise every day. Whatever you can do is fine — a swim or a short walk with a friend. If you are bedridden, stretch your toes, flex your ankles, massage your arms and legs, or just open and close your hands.

In his book, *Man's Search for Meaning*, psychiatrist Viktor E. Frankl examined the personalities of Holocaust survivors. He observed that those who had found meaning in life were more likely to have survived. Often, these hardy souls had found that being alive for someone else gave their day-to-day living a purpose. A man might think about caring for his wife; a woman might be driven to protect her children. That impetus saw them through. Similarly, patients who can't summon the enthusiasm to go on living for their own sakes might ask, "What will happen to the people I love if I leave them?"

HOW TO TAKE CONTROL OF YOUR LIFE
ଟ➥

The trauma of facing serious illness has the positive effect of forcing you to take a good look at your life. Does it seem too much of a struggle to continue? How would you change your life if you could? Once you see clearly what you don't like about your life and how you would like to change it, you will also see what you can do to bring about those changes.

Be discerning about the help you get. Family members or close friends may have great intentions, but could love you so much that they themselves become devastated by your illness and see things as hopeless. If that's the case, they can't really give you the support you need to survive. If the person trying to help you doesn't make you feel better and more hopeful, don't waste precious time. Find somebody else. A skilled psychotherapist can help you work through personal issues. Keep searching until you hook up with someone who helps you to find the courage and positivity you need.

Learning to cultivate a hopeful outlook is simple. Here are a few ways to get started. First thing in the morning, look in the bathroom mirror and tell yourself, "Good morning." Smile. Look at the curve of your lips and remember that expression. Remember what your face feels like when you smile. Good. Brush your teeth. Smile. Remember the look and feeling. Take care of your shaving, make-up, hair or wig, whatever you can do to feel well-groomed and presentable. Smile again. When you walk out of the bathroom, take the memory of the feeling and the look of your smile. Take that memory and bring it into every part of your day. Use it. When you pass a mirror, smile. If you catch yourself dragging, smile. Pull up the corners of your mouth. Think of it as a bootstrap operation.

Continue this way, thinking positively, feeling positively about yourself. At some point, it will stop feeling forced and will begin feeling genuine. Don't get discouraged if you falter along the way; acknowledge the part of you that's complaining, "This is too hard for me," then leave it behind. Don't let yourself remain in a negative state. Start again.

You may not feel happy or positive, but act happy. Recite *positive tapes*, listing the things you appreciate about yourself. Find something good that is happening in your life. It is hard to keep these thoughts in mind when you are very sick and lying in a hospital bed, waiting endlessly for your nurse to bring the pain medication. I can hear you objecting, "This is crazy. How can I feel happy and positive when I'm in pain and the outcome is bleak?" You're right, you are in a difficult spot, sick and in pain. But you can't change the pain, you can only change your attitude. Give yourself a pep talk over and over, if necessary. Tell yourself that the medication is coming and it will help. Soon I'll feel better. I can help turn my prognosis around. I can be positive. When the nurse walks in with your medication, smile at her and say, "Thanks, I know this will make me feel a lot better."

If I had to pick the most critical word among the thousands on the subject of mind-body connections, the word I would select is *hope*. That's the enabler. Maintain your belief that things can improve, then strive to make it possible.

Surround yourself with *up* people, and teach people that you need them to be optimistic for you. Unfortunately, when you are in the hospital and people come to visit you, the conversation often turns gloomy. Don't stand for that. Just cut people off with a firm, "Hey, no unpleasant conversation, please."

Celebrate every little plus. Can you keep food down after heavy vomiting? Great! That's a plus. Is your pain a little less severe than it was an hour ago? Wonderful! Once you've trained yourself to seek out the good news or signs and focus on them, your perspective will shift. You can't keep optimistic and pessimistic thoughts in your head at the same time.

Deluge yourself with positive mental *tapes*. The more you think about the good things that are happening, the more such things will happen. Developing the ability to see them is an important survival skill. You can control how you perceive things; you can work on your attitude. What have you got to lose?

Get moving.

Get help, get positive, and get well.

. . . PERSONAL PERSPECTIVE
ह⋟

Humor is one of the greatest tools I used. Often while I was on chemotherapy, I would notice my friends trying unsuccessfully not to look at my head. I knew they were thinking: "I've heard chemotherapy makes your hair fall out. I wonder. Is that a wig?"

I would pat my wig and say, "You wouldn't believe how fast my hair fell out! It all came out in great big clumps. Under this wig, I'm a female Yul Brynner!"

One Saturday, my husband and I passed under a tree as we were walking to Sabbath services. I felt a slight tug. I turned and saw my wig hanging from a low branch, swinging gently in the breeze. A few feet away, a little old lady stared at me in fascination and horror, her eyes bulging.

What could I do? I retrieved my wig, adjusted it over my bald pate, shrugged, threw my hands in the air and gave that lady my warmest smile. Sure, it was a little embarrassing. But that anecdote always brings a laugh. I've used it again and again to help cancer patients see a bit of humor in their disease or to let them have a laugh at my expense.

Another thing that worked was practicing the relaxation exercise. It helped me learn how to get in touch with my body tension. It often provided clues to my emotional state, as well. I got so good at being in touch with myself that I could tell if I was angry, fearful, anxious, sad, happy, peaceful or elevated. As a very ill cancer patient, one of my chief goals was to be in an elevated state of mind. I found that just thinking happy thoughts wasn't always enough. When I felt really low, I wasn't very successful at keeping happy thoughts foremost, so I used a behavioral approach.

Whenever I felt the corners of my mouth dragging down, it set off a flashing light in my mind. "Oh, oh, Sarah," I warned myself, "feels like you're getting low." Quickly, I made a strong effort to lift the corners of my mouth to a smile. I'd try to catch my reflection in a nearby window or mirror and view the smile. It's hard to be low with a smile on your face. Try it and you'll see. However, this only works when you make the attitude match the action. You have to want to become happy.

Combining relaxation techniques with meditation gave me a powerful means of adjusting my attitude, and a potent weapon against pain. I always connected with God in my meditation. It never failed to help. The first time I took advantage of this technique was the morning I woke up with excruciating pain racking every organ of my body. Through meditation, visualization and deep relaxation I was better able to handle the pain.

After a while, I felt as if I had left my body. I was hovering over it, looking down at it. I knew all about the dreadful pain it was experiencing. I can still recall describing it to myself as a full-blown symphony of pain that involved every fiber of my being. And yet I was detached from it. I wasn't in the pain, I was floating above it.

It was oddly, exquisitely beautiful. I have no idea how long the experience lasted, but many times since then I've been able to call upon this exercise to eliminate pain. Aside from getting me through some nasty times with cancer, meditation has become my first recourse in the dentist's chair.

I concentrated on these survival skills. I needed to continue to develop them to keep my spirits high. With elevated spirits, I was ready and able to tackle everything. I could be firm with my doctors, get the most from my nurses, and take care of my emotional and physical well-being as well.

Chapter 17

NON-TOXIC THERAPIES:
ALTERNATIVE CANCER APPROACHES

We've already discussed the traditional approaches western medicine uses to treat cancer, such as surgery, chemotherapy and radiation and other modalities. Be alert to alternative and non-toxic therapies as well, particularly nutrition and lifestyle changes.

Non-toxic therapy involves the use of anti-cancer agents that do not harm your body. This can include a healthful diet, vitamins, minerals, herbs, enzymes and other natural substances. The underlying philosophy of these therapies usually rests on restoring the immune system, dissolving cancer cells, eliminating toxins and rebuilding a strong body so the patient can maintain good health. Lifestyle alternative therapies can include developing a positive state of mind, exercise, relaxation, visualization and meditation.

I recommend you look into some of these approaches not as an anti-cancer treatment, but as a supportive adjunct to state-of-the-art medical treatment.

CONFIRMING
THE BENEFITS

In 1984, with partial funding from the National Institute of Health (NIH), Barrie R. Cassileth, Ph.D., when at the University of Pennsylvania Cancer Center, and Helene Brown, of the Jonsson Comprehensive Cancer Center at the University of California, Los Angeles, conducted an in-depth study of unorthodox, alternative or unproven cancer treatments.

They reported that cancer patients spend approximately $4 billion each year on unproven cancer cures. Middle-to-upper-class patients were most likely to seek alternative cancer therapies, and they tended to be better educated than those who had chemotherapy, radiation therapy or surgery alone.

The researchers pointed out that some alternative remedies also appear to be related to theories that are presently under aggressive conventional investigation.

The study revealed that in Great Britain one of the few growth industries is alternative medicine, which was favored by 86 percent of 100 young doctors surveyed. Great Britain is somewhat advanced in this area. England's Cancer Help Center, which offers alternative medicine in place of — or as an adjunct to — conventional cancer treatment, opened in Bristol in 1983. In keeping with the British Royal Family's use and support of alternative therapies, the Prince of Wales was on hand to open the center.

Back on our side of the Atlantic, Cassileth and Brown's report includes suggestions to clinicians. For example, they emphasize "the need to maintain open communications with the patient." (In alternative medicine, patients have an active role in their own care.) They stress that patients need to feel free to discuss alternative treatments with their oncologists without the threat of abandonment and without having an alternative approach summarily dismissed as *quackery*, with no explanation offered.

The authors view supportive psychotherapy as a helpful adjunct. A final recommendation of Cassileth and

Brown is: Conventional medicine can and should respond by incorporating the reasonable components of unorthodox therapy that patients find lacking within the traditional health care framework.

Non-traditional, non-toxic therapies vary widely. Some are very controversial and each proposal you encounter should be weighed carefully and judged sensibly, with appropriate guidance. There are many quacks and rip-off artists promoting alternative therapies. Some recommend specific foods, diets or supplements that do no good and in some cases can be harmful. Be sure you check the credentials of the *experts* connected to the therapy you consider. Check into their training and talk with patients who have been treated successfully. Any advocates of therapies mentioned in this book have had substantial education and training, have published information on their specialities, and have a body of patients who were successfully treated.

FINDING INFORMATION ON THE ALTERNATIVES
ફ✎

Many patients find John M. Fink's book *Third Opinion* very helpful. It is an international directory of alternative cancer programs and cancer support groups which includes costs and method of treatment and other relevant information about the programs in the book. The author advises his readers to request that a center substantiate its claims by citing cases that can be verified. Bear in mind that neither the author nor the publisher recommends or endorses any of the therapies. The purpose of the book is merely to provide information. The author states, "It would be wise to consult with a knowledgeable physician before undertaking a therapy."

Another book, *Crackdown On Cancer* by Ruth Yale Long, Ph.D., explains in simple language the basic theory of many of the more widely used alternative cancer therapies. The specifics of each therapy's treatment plan is included as well. The book also contains an overview of the immune system and the nutrients that are essential to build it up and to maintain good health.

The Cancer Control Society in Los Angeles (see Appendix VI) maintains a roster of recovered cancer patients who have been involved in non-toxic treatment plans, including some controversial approaches used in other countries. If you call the society at (213) 663-7801, counselors there will try to put you in touch with a patient who has recovered from the same type of cancer you have. Since evidence indicates that specific types of cancer respond more favorably than others to certain non-toxic therapies, this service could be particularly helpful.

Another informational service is the Foundation for Advancement in Cancer Therapy (FACT), Box 1242 Old Chelsea Station, New York, New York 10113, telephone: (212) 741-2790, with a chapter in Philadelphia also. Ms. Ruth Sackman, the director, reports that the only therapies considered are those that have been proved to be non-invasive, harmless, and that have been shown to help eliminate toxins and help restore and fortify the body. There is no charge for services, but contributions are accepted.

The World Research Foundation (WRF), a worldwide, non-profit health and environmental information network headquartered in Sherman Oaks, California, was established in 1984 by Steven and LaVerne Ross. For a nominal fee, you can tap into their computer search, or they will prepare for you a comprehensive packet which provides information culled from 5,000 medical journals in more than 100 countries on conventional therapies, surgery, drugs, and alternative or complementary medicine. This is certainly a nice option, not only for anyone looking for alternative therapy, but for conventional medicine as well.

When consulting a recovered patient about the success of a particular therapy, ask about related issues, such as the stage at which the cancer was checked and any other variables that may have been a factor in their improvement. I queried many recovered cancer patients throughout the United States who used non-toxic therapies and I found that all had a high degree of faith in the approach, in themselves, and in some spiritual source.

This makes me wonder if part of the success of the non-toxic therapies, when they do work, could be the strong motivation, aggressiveness and positive mindset of the patients.

Case after case in Judith Glassman's *The Cancer Survivors* underscores this point. What her examples confirm is that patients who have a positive attitude about their treatment plan are more likely to benefit from it.

O. Carl Simonton, M.D., co-author of *Getting Well Again* and head of the Simonton Cancer Center in Pacific Palisades, California, uses relaxation, visualization, exercise and a positive mindset to enhance the efficacy of state-of-the-art conventional medical treatment of cancer. Similar techniques are used by Bernie S. Siegel, M.D., author of *Love Medicine and Miracles*, who directs the Exceptional Cancer Patient Program in New Haven, Connecticut, where patients are encouraged to take control of their lives.

There are numerous support groups such as the Wellness Community of Santa Monica, California, the Wellness Center in Santa Barbara, California, the Palm Beach Wellness Center in Royal Palm Beach, Florida, and Vital Alternatives, Inc., in Sunrise, Florida, that offer support, encouragement, updates on medical treatment and care, and alternative lifestyles at no charge. To find a similar group near you, check the social services listings in the Yellow Pages, the CIS at 1-800-4-CANCER, or your local American Cancer Society.

CHANGING EATING
HABITS AND LIFESTYLES
ಬ್

I strongly urge anyone contemplating an alternative approach that involves a drastic change in eating habits, for instance, to undertake a new regimen only under the watchful eye of a physician or health care practitioner trained in nutrition. Your body is a delicately balanced machine. A sudden change in diet without supervision could be counterproductive. Sometimes switching from a traditional Western diet to a strict, unfamiliar *health food* routine may trigger a toxic reaction.

One alternative approach that I was encouraged to follow and that has received much attention is the *macrobiotic diet*. It is a diet composed primarily of whole grains, orange and green vegetables, including lots of green leafy ones, dried beans and sea vegetables, soups, a small amount of white-meat fish, cooked fruit desserts, roasted seeds, and some nuts. Beverages are mostly twig, roasted brown rice, barley, or dandelion teas and cereal grain coffee. Miso, a cultured soybean paste, is recommended for daily use, as is natural tamari soy sauce. Roasted powdered seaweed, umiboshi plum (a salted pickled plum), sesame salt, and Tekka, a vegetable paste, can be used as condiments.

It sounds quite simple, but I promise you it's not. A key to macrobiotic diets — as well as to most alternative dietary life-styles — is balance. It is crucial in the macrobiotic way of eating to consume the prescribed foods in the proper proportions, in the proper combinations, and in the proper way.

The macrobiotic diet (a diet that allows nothing artificial) is healthy, but it is totally foreign to our western habits. The foods are strange. The ways they must be prepared are strange. Following the plan takes commitment.

No one should try to become macrobiotic without strict professional supervision. This was the major drawback of the diet for me. At the time, there were very few macrobiotic counselors available.

Following the regimen requires special cooking classes, or at least a knowledgeable teacher to supervise your cooking at the beginning. Even then, it is helpful to have someone you can call for advice from time to time.

I found this non-toxic therapy to be a beneficial adjunct to the orthodox medical treatment I received, but only that. Still, cancer patients need to be aware that these other approaches exist. Some are weird and not credible. Some are far out; some are harmful. As I stated, some are quacks with fad therapies. Yet, there are non-toxic therapies that have scored some impressive victories against cancer. In this light, proper nutrition, in particular, bears deeper examination.

If you have been diagnosed with cancer, you would be remiss not to eliminate certain foods from your diet. Consider at least the foods with chemical additives, preservatives and possibly cancer-causing agents — such as high fats, alcohol, and caffeine. Cigarettes, of course, are out. If you developed cancer, that tells you that your body may have a propensity to develop it again. It may well be that something in your lifestyle, your heredity, your environment or your way of eating may have been a factor in precipitating cancer. Doesn't it make sense for you to be particularly careful about these potential sources of danger? You may not be able to do anything about heredity or your environment, but you certainly can improve your lifestyle and the way you eat.

The available knowledge is vast on both the nutritional values of foods and on how to combine them to achieve a healthy balance. The problem is discerning which dietary programs have validity and which do not; which information is accurate and which is not. Your common sense, personal research, a qualified counselor, and your physician must be your guides on those matters.

I strongly urge the cancer patients I see to adopt some form of alternative dietary and lifestyle approach in conjunction with state-of-the-art medical treatment. Some may be able to handle only part of a particular nutritional or a lifestyle therapy. That's better than nothing. Being particular about eating healthy foods is your way of saying, "I care enough about me to do my share in eating healthy and living healthy to enhance my chance of survival." It also is your way of taking an active part in your own care.

... PERSONAL PERSPECTIVE

In my struggle against malignancy, I was willing to look into anything that might take me a step closer to victory. However, when it came to nutrition, I found that the dietary approaches with the best track records were outside the mainstream of modern medical thought.

When I was undergoing chemotherapy, I consulted the head dietitian at a very reputable hospital who gave me a booklet published by a protein supplement manufacturer that stressed lots of calories in the forms of milk shakes, ice cream, custards, steaks, snacks of potato chips, pretzels, chocolate cake. I wondered if the dietary recommendations could possibly have been written with my best interests in mind.

I threw the booklet away and even though I had only a layman's knowledge, I knew its advice was all wrong. However, the experience pushed me to think about eating in a more healthy way. A friend recommended that I carefully explore a macrobiotic diet.

I did. Nutritionally it made a lot of sense to me. I followed an exceedingly rigid macrobiotic medicinal recommendation. I think it helped. As I had more chemotherapy treatments, I became increasingly weaker — yet after I started the macrobiotic diet three months into my treatment, I began to feel stronger. My energy level increased. I felt better and my blood counts remained within normal range. Common sense told me something must have been supporting my immune system — and I knew it wasn't the chemotherapy. I continued my chemotherapy but also remained macrobiotic.

Some of the things I learned were:

(1) Soaking grains overnight makes them easier to digest;

(2) Don't eat for three hours before going to sleep;

(3) Collard greens are an excellent source of calcium;

(4) Sugar depletes calcium;

(5) It's crucial to combine a certain quantity of legumes with grains to get a complete protein.

(6) Cancer patients need to chew all grains 100 times because digestion of grains begins with the digestive juices of the mouth.

Several years after I completed chemotherapy and was not so rigidly macrobiotic, a helpful suggestion from a macrobiotic adviser was that when I'd binge and eat pizza, ice cream or whatever, I should simply take an herbal laxative before I went to sleep to quickly eliminate the harmful by-products.

I take acidophilus, a cultured product, when a doctor prescribes an antibiotic for me. Acidophilus is effective in increasing the healthy bacteria in the intestine.

In all, I have instituted the following alternative therapies and lifestyle changes:

(1) Relaxation exercises
(2) Exercise program
(3) Macrobiotic diet (with some digressions)
(4) Vitamin and mineral supplements
(5) Changing my attitude to one of greater assertiveness
(6) Enhanced spirituality

I credit these lifestyle changes as being a strong factor in having survived my cancer, having a more positive outlook and with my current state of remission and good health.

Chapter 18

NUTRITION ALERT:
DIET AWARENESS CAN HELP YOU WIN

Until recently, nutrition has been a neglected area in modern medicine. A brilliant cancer surgeon once told me, "You seem to know a lot more about nutrition than I do. We only had one course in it in medical school." But that picture is changing.

Based on scientific studies, the American Institute for Cancer Research in Washington, D.C. reports that the best estimate of all cancer deaths attributed to dietary factors is 30 percent and might extend as high as 70 percent. The Institute invites you to dial 1-800-843-8114 to access their Nutrition and Cancer Hot Line.

WHAT YOU EAT
CAN HELP
&

Recent research at some cancer centers confirms the nutritional value of certain foods in preventing some cancers as well as a recurrence of cancer. One nutrient is the subject of a study initiated by Dr. Ann Kennedy, when she was a radiobiologist at the Harvard School of Public Health. She is studying *protease inhibitors*, which are nontoxic anti-cancer agents. One, in particular, a protease inhibitor derived from soybeans, is the subject of a five-to-ten-year study to observe its effects on head and neck cancers. Dr. Kennedy continues her work at the Department of Radiation Oncology at the University of Pennsylvania.

She emphasizes that protease inhibitors are not a cure, but may prove to be a preventive measure to lower the risk of recurrence. She thinks that vitamin E and C derivatives will also prove effective.

Meanwhile, information reported by Michele Donley of Chicago in the September 2, 1991, issue of *Time* magazine delivered a strong warning that protease inhibitors in soybeans have been linked to the development of pancreatic cancer. In answer to my query, I was told that when the soybeans are heated to a certain point, the cancer-carrying agents of the soybeans are destroyed. When contraindications such as these are reported and "should I or shouldn't I" decisions need to be made, it's important to keep in mind that going it alone could sometime be harmful. This is why I repeatedly urge you not to go on any dietary program without medical advice and/or qualified supervision.

In the same article, it is reported that animal studies indicated that isoflavones in soybeans have been shown to prevent liver cancer. It pays to keep your eye on those soybeans.

Physicians have indeed found that diet is a factor in cancer. This theory is borne out by researchers' observations that prevalent forms of cancer vary from country to country according to national diet. One example of this is the low occurrence of breast cancer in the women of Japan where the national diet is relatively low in fat. Yet when Japanese women moved to the West and adopted a high-fat, Western diet, their incidence of breast cancer increased.

The Dade County (Florida) Chapter of the American Cancer Society funded a study of cancer in Hispanics, who have the lowest rates of most types of cancer. For example, pre-existing data show that there is a much lower incidence of breast and colon cancer among Hispanics than Anglos or blacks. This finding is attributed to the cultural factor of the traditional low-fat, high-fiber diet of Hispanics.

The National Cancer Institute recently started a chemoprevention program that includes a study of anti-carcinogenic foods and supplements. The relatively new American Institute for Cancer Research is also conducting investigations into dietary factors in relationship to cancer. Many cancer centers, among them the Virginia Regional Cancer Center, the University of Pennsylvania, and the University of Arizona, are researching nutrition as a cancer prevention factor.

It is encouraging to see major medical facilities take an interest in the role of diet in the cause, prevention and treatment of cancer. For instance, some hospitals are beginning to include nutrition training in their programs for cancer patients. One example is the patient diet used at American International Hospital in Zion, Illinois, which tells the patient that, *"A prudent diet is the first line of defense against cancer."*

At American International Hospital, a physician-directed diet program, uses a high-fiber menu of fresh vegetables and fruits to augment the patient's immune system. As soon as patients are admitted to the hospital, their individual nutritional needs are assessed. Doctors use sophisticated equipment to quickly determine the levels of all the constituents of the patient's immune system. This equipment can also determine whether the patient's digestive system functions properly. If it doesn't, enzymes — or other appropriate supplements — are prescribed. It is important to help patients achieve proper digestion because even the healthiest diet in the world won't help if the digestive system isn't working to take nutrients to the cells where they belong.

Each patient receives a diet plan for the duration of his or her hospital stay. Vitamins, minerals and other supplements are used when necessary. In patients' meals, honey and fructose replace white sugar. Minimal amounts of red meat are offered, and only whole-grain breads are served. No artificial colorings or preservatives are used. If needed, the hospital offers a special vegetarian diet of organically grown foods. Patients are taught how to continue their diets at home.

This is the wave of the future, I believe, particularly since the National Cancer Institute (NCI) is actively studying the role of diet in cancer.

In a March, 1988, general statement, the NCI reported that six studies are being conducted to examine the role of micronutrients and diet in preventing colon cancer. Calcium, beta-carotene, wheat bran and vitamins C and E are being studied. Other studies focus on folic acid/vitamin B12, retinol, 13-cis retinoic acid, beta-carotene, and vitamin E in the prevention of lung cancer.

At Memorial Sloan-Kettering Cancer Center, investigators are exploring ways in which diet has an impact on cancer. In recent years, the National Polyp Study, a multicenter study led by Memorial Sloan-Kettering, has helped to establish the role of dietary factors in colorectal cancer — for example, that diet influences the development of abnormalities of the lining of the bowel.

Georgetown University Medical Center reports an active clinical and research program in nutritional support. Studies of how to improve nutrition are under way at the Mayo CCC where researchers have found that well-nourished patients tend to tolerate treatments better. They respond more positively, recuperate more quickly, and feel better in general.

The Summer/Fall, 1988, issue of *OncoNews*, the Columbia University Comprehensive Cancer Center newsletter, reported the award of $6.5 million from the Lucille P. Mackey Charitable Trust to support an innovative five-year research program to study how certain environmental chemicals and dietary factors can interact with host genetic factors to cause cancer and other diseases or disorders.

Dr. Bruce Ames, a professor of cell biology at the University of California at Berkeley has for many years been an investigator of possible carcinogenic properties in various foods. Dr. Ames is the creator of the widely used

Ames Test that can identify carcinogenic potential in certain chemicals or substances found in foods. The test is said to be 90 percent accurate. Any results published about the Ames Test are worthy of our attention.

Dana-Farber Cancer Institute's newsletter offered an informative article on nutrition and cancer. It reported that "a diet high in fiber may be a factor in lowering the risk of developing colon and rectal cancers."

Fiber helps move waste materials, including chemical compounds, more rapidly through the large intestine and out of the body. Researchers suggest that there is a risk of possible damage to the intestinal tissues if these by-products and chemicals remain in the intestines too long. The rapid elimination of digestive wastes may reduce the risk of damage to the intestine and thereby reduce the risk of cancer.

Many alternative diet therapies are also based on the theory that waste materials and toxic chemicals that remain in the intestines interfere with proper digestion, thus causing damage to the body. This new wisdom has been espoused by alternative therapy experts for years.

"Poor diets are deadly," warned former U.S. Surgeon General C. Everett Koop in a front-page newspaper article in 1986. He was issuing a report cautioning Americans that "what they eat and drink is killing them."

Koop's 750-page report, which reviewed more than 2,000 studies conducted over four years, indicated that diets high in fats contribute to some types of cancer. One health official commended the report for solidifying the links between diet and health but criticized it for being too vague. He doubted that anyone would pay attention to the report because it gave no specifics on how much of any given food was too much.

Conversely, much of the appeal of the dietary alternative treatments is their specificity. They prescribe exact quantities of each type of food and each supplement. Counselors spend a lot of time explaining the reasons behind their suggestions. They encourage individuals to learn about and understand their programs and the rationale behind them.

With the alternative therapies, you become an important part of the team fighting your illness. Most cancer patients who ask their doctors about nutrition are told, "Just eat a balanced diet." But educated, inquisitive cancer patients are drawn to alternative therapies — in conjunction with standard medical treatment — because they believe that the counselors directing these treatments are knowledgeable about balancing foods and prescribing an exact, healthy way to eat.

LEARNING ABOUT
VITAMINS AND NUTRIENTS

Vitamins and other nutrients are also important to the cancer patient, who needs sound advice on the subject from a qualified source. Exhaustive information is available from the National Academy of Sciences, publishers of *Recommended Dietary Allowances* — the *RDA*. The Academy's National Research Council has published *On Diet, Nutrition and Cancer*, a pioneering report which combines an evaluation of dietary studies and a series of guidelines based on its evaluative findings.

A useful reference book is *The Nutritional Almanac*, co-authored by John D. Kirschmann and Lavon J. Dunne. You can also garner information about almost every nutrient available. A handy book to take along with you when food shopping is *The Food Bible* by Jayne Benkendorf. It tells you what you need to know nutritionally about preservatives, additives, fats and more that are found in the items on the shelves in the market.

Vitamins A, C (with the following cautions), E and selenium are strongly recommended for cancer patients.

Vitamin A is found in carrots and other yellow-orange-colored foods that are rich in beta-carotene, which is believed to have anti-cancer effects. Most of the alternative cancer treatments use large amounts of these yellow-orange foods. Some programs use a lot of carrot juice in particular. Natural vitamin A (beta-carotene) sources include liver, fish liver oil, eggs, certain dairy products and yellow-orange vegetables,

carrots and green vegetables and fruits. Too much syn-
thetic vitamin A can cause problems — not more than
10,000 IU's (International Units) should be taken.

Vitamin C, found in citrus fruits, berries and green
and leafy vegetables as well as cauliflower, helps restore
the immune system, which becomes depressed by chemotherapy. But when taken with manganese and copper,
vitamin C can generate free-radicals, which are generally
believed to be cancer-producing. In addition to other conditions, too much vitamin C may be harmful for patients
being evaluated for colon cancer. Patients receiving
methotrexate should not take vitamin C when getting
infusions, although they may take it between treatments.

Linus Pauling, two-time winner of the Nobel Prize,
and Ewan Cameron advocate high dosages of vitamin C
between treatments, but they tell patients to refrain from
vitamin C for 24 to 48 hours following chemotherapy
treatments. Many in the field of medicine, however, disagree with Pauling's high-dose vitamin C therapy.

Some researchers indicate that it is possible to determine how much vitamin C is appropriate for your system
by gradually increasing the dosage until you have one loose
stool. This indicates your bowel tolerance and is your
signal to reduce the dosage.

Vitamin E is thought to act to prevent cancer and is
beneficial in fibrocystic disease of the breast. According to
experimental data, patients can benefit from vitamins C
and E during radiation therapy. Vitamin E, found in dried
beans, green leafy vegetables, liver, vegetable oils, wheat
germ, and whole grain cereals and whole wheat flour, is
known to be an important factor in stimulating the immune system. This helps reduce cancer risks.

Selenium seeks out and destroys free-radicals, which
are believed to be cancer producing. Foods rich in selenium
are chicken, egg yolks, garlic, meat, milk, seafood, onions,
broccoli as well as whole-grain cereals, such as wheat
germ, and bran. Selenium and vitamin E taken together
have a stronger effect. They are synergistic, the whole
being greater than its parts.

Calcium is an important mineral found in broccoli, salmon, cheese, sunflower seeds, green vegetables, dried beans, soybeans, peas, milk, sardines, yogurt and sesame. However, cancer patients with bone metastasis should not take supplementary calcium without consulting their physicians.

Indole-3 Carbinol. On June 6, 1990, *The Miami Herald* reported a Reuters News Service item that H. Leon Bradlow of the Institute for Hormone Research in New York City and his colleague Jon J. Michnovicz had identified a chemical, indole-3 carbinol, which is found in cruciferous vegetables, and which they believe reduces the risk of breast cancer. Cruciferous vegetables include cabbage, broccoli, cauliflower, and Brussels sprouts. Their results confirm previous studies that found lower cancer rates among people whose diets were rich in cabbage and broccoli, including Chinese and Korean women. Dr. Bradlow told me that studies in people and animals showed that administration of indole-3 carbinol alters estrogen metabolism to produce a less potent compound. This altered metabolite pattern of estrogens serves to block the development of breast cancer in mice. (Now in press.)

Glucarate. A May 11, 1990, article in the *Jewish Press*, a weekly newspaper, reported another study involving the cruciferous vegetables. Zbigniew Walaszek, Ph.D., a biochemist at University of Texas System Cancer Center with the help of a grant from the American Institute for Cancer Research in Washington, D.C., has tested glucarate, a salt of glucaris acid which is found naturally in broccoli, Brussels sprouts, bean sprouts, cauliflower, and other plant foods. Laboratory studies indicated that glucarate seems to prevent the development of cancer. Tumor growth in laboratory animals seems to slow substantially even when glucarate is given after a cancer develops. Tumors that appear to be inhibited by glucarate are those of the lungs, skin, liver, colon, and particularly those of the breasts.

Glucarate is not available in pill form, so it might be a good idea to develop a taste for broccoli, cabbage and other cruciferous vegetables.

HARMFUL FOODS AND
DRINKS — WATCH OUT!

ॐ

A higher incidence of cancers of the breast, thyroid, oral cavity, respiratory track and malignant melanoma are associated with the use of alcohol. A higher incidence of breast cancer is associated with high-fat diets, as was borne out at a breast cancer symposium in January, 1989, at Columbia-Presbyterian Medical Center where the late Dr. Angelos Papatestis, of Mount Sinai Medical Center in New York City, reported on "Obesity-Risk and Prognosis."

Our environment and what we eat, drink and smoke, some studies suggest, may account for as much as 80 percent of all cancers. This has influenced the American Cancer Society to start a health awareness program for the 1990's called the *Great American Food Fight Against Cancer*. The ACS plans to bring to the attention of schools, businesses, supermarkets and restaurants the relationship between diet and cancer as well as to inform the public of what constitutes a healthy way of eating.

A 1990 revision on *Suggestions On Nutrition And Nutritional Supplements* from the Cancer Research Institute in New York City advised, *"Three* studies are now showing an *increased* risk of prostate cancer with increased ingestion of carotene."* When I read something like this and it is from a credible institution, I suggest to prostate cancer patients they hold up on carrot juices and squash soups until all the facts are in.

Vitamins, minerals, and the like, while classified as non-toxic because they do not damage the immune system, are not necessarily benign. Thus, for general health care, I would recommend a physician whose speciality is preventive medicine. Unlike the average medical doctor who spends approximately thirty hours in the study of nutrition during his medical training, physicians who specialize in preventive medicine have had extensive training in nutrition, vitamin and mineral therapy and exercise. Doctors who specialize in preventive medicine also have experience in building up and restoring the immune system.

Because vitamins are readily available, and anticancer drugs are not, you may be tempted to experiment. Don't. You need consistent professional monitoring of your body's warnings if you are to increase your chances of survival. It is also important to work with a professional so that you feel confident about the treatment you get.

. . . PERSONAL PERSPECTIVE

One problem I have found with many anti-cancer agents is that their effects are temporary. When the patient discontinues them, they stop working and the cancer cells return. Evidence exists, as you have read, that protease inhibitors appear to stop the recurrence of some cancers. This suggests to me that the two daily bowls of macrobiotic miso soup, high in protease inhibitors, which I drank religiously for three or four years during and after my conventional cancer treatment, may have been a factor in non-recurrence of my cancer. I think another factor was the seaweeds, cruciferous vegetables, greens and other foods I ate on the macrobiotic diet which were full of high doses of the vitamins, minerals and other substances which have been discussed in this chapter as having cancer prevention potential.

Although a strict macrobiotic diet permits no vitamin or mineral supplements, I took vitamins C and E on the advice of a physician. These vitamins have demonstrated an effect on cancer, so I can conclude that they, too, may have been part of the reason why my lymphoma has not recurred.

Today, I continue to follow many of the recommendations of macrobiotic eating, but I am not as rigid about it as I was when I was ill. However, because of my involvement with this diet, I did a lot of research and learned a great deal about the nutritional factor in cancer treatment. Today, I eat sensibly and avoid foods that might be carcinogenic and those with chemical additives. I have come to think of nutritional therapy as another important spoke in the wheel of cancer treatment.

Chapter 19

BUILDING YOUR TEAM:
LET YOUR FAMILY (FRIENDS, SUPPORT GROUP) FIGHT CANCER WITH YOU

The support you need as you battle cancer can come from many different sources — your family, your friends, professionals and volunteer support organizations. If it is hard to reach out, start with the people closest to you, your immediate family and close friends. They can help so much, practically and emotionally. Everyone has something special to offer.

When you're not feeling well, practical things become difficult: getting to and from the doctor's office, filling out hospital forms, cooking, cleaning. Family and friends can help you cope with the nitty-gritty aspects of daily life, with medical decisions, with financial worries.

Most precious of all is the intangible, emotional support they give, as anyone who has suffered a serious illness will tell you. The moments of intimate communication mean the most, the times when the bittersweet bond of love and anguish between stricken patient and loving parent, mate or child finds expression. It may be no more than an arm around the shoulder, but the gesture says, "I love you and I'm here."

The other side of the coin are those who don't have

family or friends. Unfortunately, there are many. If you are alone, alert the members of your religious community of your needs. They can be very supportive and caring. In fact, you may go from having no one to acquiring a large, extended family. Religious community members can help with everyday tasks, such as shopping, marketing and meals. There may even be those who are willing to drive you to your treatments or doctor's appointments. Even if you haven't been in a synagogue, temple or church in years, if you call a rabbi, minister or priest and state your case, you'll get help. And you don't have to make a commitment to their cause. Of course, they would like that, too, but they take people *as is*, with no questions asked. Help is there for you, but you have to let your needs be known.

LETTING OTHERS HELP

ȝ☙

As the cancer profile indicates, people who get cancer tend to drive themselves hard and to have trouble expressing needs, feelings and frustrations. You may find it hard to ask for help, but help is there. You can bear up bravely and avoid being a burden without being a martyr.

You may try to shield loved ones by keeping them in ignorance of the true nature of your disease. In many cases, you do yourself and your loved ones a disservice. When the truth comes out, as it is almost always bound to, the person you tried to protect will have to deal with hurt feelings as well as with the shock of knowing you have cancer. You are depriving him or her of caring for you and expressing love at a time when you need that love and care very much.

Many times in counseling I've heard the anguish of a parent — a grown child, brother or sister or spouse who was devastated for years after a family member's death at not having been told the extent of the illness until it was too late. The pain of not having the opportunity to rectify past misunderstandings or merely to say, "I love you," was not easy for the relative to bear. Some family members simply want the chance to say, "Goodbye."

HEALTHY FAMILIES MAKE
HEALTHIER PATIENTS

Studies have shown that sometimes seemingly happy families are more easily shattered by catastrophic illness. Since their family life always went smoothly, they didn't acquire well-practiced methods of dealing with extreme stress. I saw an example of this when I walked into a hospital room to find the highly-educated wife of a very successful lawyer angrily berating her critically ill husband. She was livid with resentment that he'd let her down by getting sick! Families like this, who don't get help, often end up as broken families where one member or several live with very guilty feelings for years down the line.

Meeting the various needs of an immediate family member causes cancer patients a great deal of anxiety. High on the list is the question of fulfilling a spouse's sexual needs. Certainly, many people look to sexual intimacy as a source of enjoyment and comfort all through their cancer treatments. But when a patient is feeling zapped out, nauseated and half-dead, sex is not uppermost in mind.

I've heard from many patients that they participated sexually at the cost of great pain and exhaustion. I think it is up to the healthy spouse to show consideration. If a patient doesn't have the energy to make it through the day doing the minimal things necessary to survive, it doesn't seem fair to rob them of what little energy they have. It's not difficult to know whether a person's energy is flagging. Just test with a few tentative advances and see what the response is.

Men who are facing sterility from certain surgeries, chemotherapies and radiation can have sperm deposited into a sperm bank. Women of child-bearing age can discuss with their physicians what options they have with regard to having children. Some people may think they have a problem with this with respect to their religious beliefs and may want to check with their clergy prior to making such decisions.

These things need to be talked about and resolved

with mutual respect and understanding. These are sensitive subjects, and every couple needs to come to terms with them in their own way.

A patient may also feel stress about a spouse's social needs. Most of us can push beyond our limits a little bit, and sometimes that extra effort may even be good for us. But you have to be aware of just how far you can go. First, respect the demands of your own body.

If you are a cancer patient with young children, you have to make it clear exactly what you can do. If you don't speak up, your family will expect a more-or-less normal level of participation. Remember, nobody else knows what's going on inside you, including your feelings of resentment, loss and frustration as well as weakness and pain. This needs to be expressed so that arrangements for such things as child care can be made. Try to make a little personal quiet time for each child and remember: the most important thing you can do for your children is to work at getting well.

When a child has cancer, the support of the family — especially the mother — is all-important. She sets the tone. She must be careful to maintain a positive attitude. Children's sensitivity to the moods of the adults around them is well known. Every effort should be made to keep the atmosphere cheerful. But too much pampering can send a negative message. That, along with a woeful, anxious expression, may give the child the message that he or she is very sick and might even die. The same signals will be picked up by other children in the family, and they will reinforce the patient's preoccupation with death. The best approach is to carry on as before, as much as possible, holding firm to a positive attitude.

Affording you some kind of respite is also something your family can provide. They allow you to take time to regroup and heal after you've completed your treatment. As time goes by, you will want to venture out a bit. You will feel more rested and more in control. The warmth, the love, the caring will make you whole again. This is the special magic of family love.

HOSPITAL VISITS

Remember to let your friends know that you need their friendship now, more than ever. When people are stricken with a serious illness such as cancer, and particularly when they're hospitalized, friends often stay away to avoid taxing the patient's strength. They don't want to impose. This is a common misunderstanding. Emotionally healthy patients, when asked if they are up to a visit, usually respond, "Positively! I want my friends to come. I don't want to feel abandoned!"

There is nothing to stop you, the patient, from taking the initiative. If you are feeling lonely, pick up the phone and call a friend. You can suggest that a visit would be welcome without putting your friend on the spot. Ask for a particular book, a magazine, some stationery — whatever would be appropriate — if your friend has a chance to come by. If you feel uncomfortable about calling, have a family member call for you. Let your friends know that you would like to see them.

Visitors need to be mindful, though, of what they talk about. I've had many cancer patients tell me how painful it was to listen to other people ramble on about things like how rough a time they are having with a co-worker or how much pain they feel from the sprained ankle they have, and all the while the patient wanted to yell, "Hey, look at me, calmly sitting here listening to your insignificant complaints when my life is on the line. I've got cancer! I just had surgery! I'm getting radiation! I hurt! I'm scared!"

It's okay to let someone know if you want to change the conversation or if you are too tired for conversation. Few guests realize that they can come and just sit quietly. A visitor can always bring a book along and say, "If it's all right, I'll just sit and read a bit. If you feel like talking, let me know and I'd be happy to chat. If you don't, that's okay, too."

The simple fact of having someone present comforts the patient. *Visiting means caring.* It rekindles hope and determination. If family and friends ask what they can do, tell them, "Come see me."

This is not a blanket prescription for visiting cancer patients. There are times when visitors are an invasion of the patient's privacy. You need to be sensitive to the wishes of the patients and their families. It's always appropriate to call first.

HOSPICE PROGRAM

ह~

I find that many patients who qualify for hospice, and their families, are not familiar with how the program works. In electing a hospice program, a patient opts for pain control and to be kept as comfortable as possible and agrees to forgo any further medical treatment or experimental programs or life-support systems. If the hospice is certified by Medicare, the patient also relinquishes Medicare coverage in favor of full hospice services, which are paid for by the hospice program. Patients who are under 65 years and meet the criteria can become eligible for Medicare. That would qualify them for the hospice program.

The hospice program, in turn, provides at no charge home care, including house cleaning and laundry, nursing care, pastoral counselors, social workers, nursing home counseling, and anticipatory grieving. To qualify a patient for hospice, the doctor must declare that the patient is terminally ill and has six months or less to live. There must be a caregiver in the home, or the patient can go to the home of a friend or to a nursing home.

The chief goal of hospice is to keep the patient free of pain and as comfortable as possible. Though the hospice program is geared to home care, a patient is still eligible for hospital care if the following criteria are met:

1. uncontrolled pain; need more skilled care or more sophisticated equipment and medications.
2. intractable nausea, vomiting, diarrhea, bed sores that might require monitoring and care by registered nurses.
3. respite for family; 4-5 days of hospitalization permitted.
4. active phase of dying; patient does not want to

die at home. Patient and/or the family would feel more confidence and comfort in a hospital environment where physicians and nurses are available at all times.

If a patient seeks medical care for a heart problem or surgery for gallbladder or something else not provided by the program, or if the patient hears of a new experimental trial for his type of cancer and wishes to avail himself of it, it is possible to leave hospice by signing a revocation form. The patient is thus reinstated into Medicare. If after the medical care and/or surgery, or if the effects of the investigational treatment are not effective, and if the patient later wants to re-enter the hospice program, a physician need merely again sign the forms that qualify him.

JOIN THE CLUB: SUPPORT FROM ORGANIZATIONS

The support you need may begin with your family and then your friends, but it doesn't stop there. Organized support groups, particularly those where you are in contact with recovered cancer patients, can provide tremendous bolstering and assistance.

"If I could only have seen a person who had recovered from lung cancer, it would have meant everything to me. If he never said a word, I would still know that if he could do it, I could do it too," explains Richard Bloch, a recovered patient mentioned in Chapter 4 who went on to establish a cancer support foundation, which is noted for its hot line manned by recovered cancer patients (see Appendix VI). His heartfelt words might have been spoken by any one of the millions of people who have faced cancer.

Support groups exist in such variety that even defining the term is difficult. Any group that responds to one of the seemingly inexhaustible needs of cancer patients qualifies as a support group, be it your family, a hospital-based peer group, a community-based or national group, a religious group, or your friends.

Often groups of cancer patients bonded by their common struggle can provide each other with excellent short-term or long-term emotional support. Such groups are sponsored by hospitals, non-profit organizations, national societies, and religious organizations. Because so much depends on your ability to maintain a positive attitude, be sure the support group you chose is right for you. You can find the right one by checking with the CIS (1-800-4-CANCER), social services in the yellow pages, cancer centers and hospitals, which often have in-house support groups. Family members or doctors, all with the best intentions, may try to sell a patient on a particular group. Don't be talked into something you feel unsure about. Only you know which choices will make you comfortable — religious or secular, group or individual support — so participate actively in the decision. Look for the type of support you believe will be the most fulfilling and helpful to you.

Many social service organizations are equipped to help you deal with the nitty-gritty details of coping — transportation, home care, even wigs! Doctors may not think (or know) to tell you about such resources, so do some research yourself. If you don't know where to start, contact the American Cancer Society office nearest you. This is probably the most extensive nationwide network of support groups. They have a variety of self-help counseling, assistance and rehabilitative programs that are described in Appendix VI.

In this same Appendix, you will find additional resources. Many more can be accessed through the yellow pages and the CIS (1-800-4-CANCER).

Support and informational societies are listed in the appendix with a brief overview of the services offered.

Most of the many wish fulfillment groups for children with life-threatening or chronic illnesses are local and grant a wish that can be filled in their own community, such as dinner at a restaurant or passes to a sports or cultural event. Other groups provide patients and a family member or members a trip to a specific place such as Disneyland or Disney World.

Appendix VI lists a few groups that grant a wish to children from any area and that operate on a national or international level. Of those, Arthur Stein of Children's Wish Foundation International reported no limitations on the fulfillment as long as the wish is that of the child and is reasonable and feasible. Examples of wishes they have granted were to swim with the dolphins, to meet a celebrity, and to provide a child and his family with a festive reunion with an immediate family member who was flown in from the Middle East. Some of these groups are more limited than others in the wishes that they grant and have more stringent requirements for a child to qualify. I suggest you query more than one group.

Summer camps for children with cancer and related illnesses abound. You need to make an application early since most camps are for one- or two-week sessions in the summer and spaces may be taken up quickly.

In Appendix VI, you will be told how to find these camps and a few with some unique programs are listed.

One of these camps founded by Paul Newman is The Hole-In-The-Wall-Gang Camp (THITWGC). A special feature of the camp is that beside the regular sessions, they have a parent retreat during the camp's fall and spring escape-week-ends, and the winterized camp facilities are available during the off-season for a variety of educational programs, seminars, and conferences for health care professionals.

At another camp, Jan Johnson, the contact person for Camp Star Trails, University of Texas, M. D. Anderson Memorial Hospital and Tumor Institute, reported they accept children with AIDS into the same camp program as the regular campers. More on these camps and others in Appendix VI.

In many communities, United Way or Community Chest also has an information and referral office. I even found some support group meetings listed in the calendar of events in my local newspaper. I received help from an organization affiliated with the Jewish faith, but non-religious groups and organizations sponsored by other denominations offer similar programs.

Community groups may also be able to help. For example, La Liga Contra El Cancer (The League Against Cancer) in Miami, Florida, a private non-profit organization, has raised millions of dollars to provide funds and free medical care to needy cancer patients since 1975. In 1987 alone, La Liga helped as many as 1,500 patients and more than 20,000 patients to date have benefited. Most of them were Hispanics, but this is an example of a group dedicated to serving a particular segment of the population. Be sure to find out if you qualify for services provided specifically to members of your nationality, profession, religion or ethnic group.

ROFEH (Reaching Out For Emergency Help), the group which helped me, is a patient/medical referral and support organization headed by Rabbi Levi I. Horowitz of Boston. It has an international reputation for offering assistance and emotional and financial support to the critically ill from all over the world. Two floors of his New England Chassidic Center on Beacon Street in Brookline are set up to accommodate patients being treated in the Boston area. Apartments in a four-story brownstone two doors down the street are available to patients' families or to individuals from great distances who have to remain for extended treatment. In addition, the Rabbi opens his nearby home to more patients. Because of his efforts, observant Jews have a place to stay where kosher dietary laws are observed and where they have access to a synagogue.

In Brooklyn, New York, other Jewish organizations that help the sick include the Rifkah Laufer and Bubov Bikor Cholim (Helping The Sick), to name a few. They have dozens of volunteers providing food, shelter, medical referrals, interpreters, medical liaisons, and even financial assistance. To find a Bikor Cholim Society in your community, check under Social Services in the yellow pages or ask your local rabbi.

For those who think they are all alone in their bout with cancer, as you have read, there is lots of help out there.

. . . PERSONAL PERSPECTIVE
ॐ

All my life, I've enjoyed being a giver. I was a listening post, always ready to lend a sympathetic ear to others while keeping my own feelings submerged. Suddenly, I found myself overwhelmed by a devastating disease that could not be pushed aside and ignored. At first, all I could do was feel sorry for myself. Fortunately, my family helped me pull myself together and redirect my limited energy toward finding ways to cope.

How easy it is to take your family for granted! I don't think I realized until much later what my husband went through during my illness, how he suffered with me. He was always there. Seymore was an unwavering source of comfort and strength as were my boys, who were in their early teens when I learned I had cancer. The spiritual books my eldest, Yehuda, brought me were just what I needed to help rally my spirits. My younger son, Jeff, so gentle and sensitive, would stick his head in my room when he came home from school and say, "Hi, Ma! How's it goin'?" The caring in his voice lifted me to great heights. My sons were one of my main reasons for living, a reason to fight, my window to hope.

When my cancer was first diagnosed, my brother, sisters and I decided to keep this knowledge from our mother. We thought it would be too much for her to handle. We told her a half-truth, that I was having thyroid surgery. But when my cancer returned and I started chemotherapy, I had to reconsider. Because she would see the side effects, the hair loss, the weakness, we decided to tell her the whole truth after my first infusion.

As we anticipated, she went to pieces. But we never anticipated her deep hurt at having been excluded from what we, as a family, were going through, her pain at not being permitted to share our heartache and our prayers.

The list of those who went out of their way to assist and support me is endless. Every day my brother Morty called and delivered to me a daily dose of spiritual infusion. My sisters, Raynah and Shelley, who both had growing families and lived out of state, never hesitated to rush to my side. They strengthened my hope and determination.

My good friend Gloria Bierman used to call me daily, offering help of any kind. When I refused it, she simply persisted until she wore me down.

When I felt as though I couldn't face another chemotherapy treatment, my dear friend of many years, Bernice Schwartz, appeared at the rabbi's home and drove me to the Dana-Farber Cancer Institute and stayed with me through the infusion. The outpouring of well-wishers was endless. The constant support did much to keep my spirits elevated.

Child or adult, the most beautiful thing a cancer patient's family and friends can do is to be there.

Chapter 20

FAITH:
A POWERFUL WEAPON

THE EPILOGUE
ح

To the One Above,
Please, God, let me be tolerant of all those
around me who love me, with all the suffering
I'm going through. Also, help me to overcome
my illness. May my hope in You give me the
strength and courage to go on. Please restore
me to health. May God bless all those people
who have been praying for me, who have given
me the strength to go on.

[A prayer placed in the Western Wall in Jerusalem
by Deborah, a young lung cancer patient.]

Faith transcends all barriers. You are never hopeless
when you have faith: faith that you'll be able to manage
whatever comes your way. It is what helps you persevere
in the face of a dire outcome. Faith can manifest itself in
trust in your ability to carry on — that your family and
friends will stand by you — or that your doctor and other

members of your health care team will be there for you to help ease your pain and provide comfort.

THE VALUE OF FAITH

Until recently, spirituality had no place in serious medical texts. Yet in spite of skepticism from the medical profession, the phenomenon of faith moving medical mountains has stubbornly persisted. There are many accounts of terminally ill patients whose doctors had given up on them, who had nothing going for them but determined faith, and who suddenly went into remission. Because of these perplexing cases, some doctors are taking another look at the role of spirituality in healing.

Dr. Herbert Benson, a prominent cardiologist and an associate professor of medicine on the staff of Harvard Medical School, after researching his *Beyond The Relaxation Response*, came to the inescapable conclusion that relaxation techniques coupled with faith have a far greater impact than relaxation techniques alone. This may be because his patients were linking meditation — which was new to them — with something familiar, comforting and trustworthy.

Faith is very real. It kicks in whenever we place utter trust in something. That "something" may vary from person to person. It may be a higher power, a doctor, a treatment plan, or one's own self. Whatever form it takes, it is the underpinning of daily life.

Essentially, belief or faith seems to connect you to the survivor within yourself. Dr. Bernie Siegel, author of *Love, Medicine and Miracles*, calls this the "inner helper." I see it as that spark of Godliness we call the soul, a powerhouse of life-giving energy.

YOUR QUALITY OF LIFE

Not everyone who has strong belief will overcome cancer, although many studies do indicate that such patients tend to survive longer. Still, some will inevitably die of the disease. But the quality of their lives, up to the final moments, is transformed and enhanced by the power of faith.

There is an unmistakable glow about people who are spiritually elevated. The *high* they feel when connected to God is beyond what I imagine any addict might experience. And their joy isn't dependent on anything outside of themselves.

The experience of tapping into the spiritual reserve within you makes you feel like a giant. When you are feeling that connection you are invincible. Nothing — literally nothing — can hurt you. Many people have this experience during life-threatening situations.

Dr. Elisabeth Kübler-Ross' book, *On Death and Dying*, is a landmark study of the near-death experience. Her subjects in this and other writings run the gamut of religious backgrounds and personal beliefs. But their reports of what they experienced on the threshold of death are remarkably similar. They speak of a sensation of floating upward, of a tunnel of light that seems to beckon. It is a euphoric experience, and some even expressed regret that they had to return to their mundane lives.

Catastrophic illness has a way of making it important for us to search for meaning in our existence. It is very common for terminal patients to turn to spirituality in search for such meaning.

In *Beyond The Relaxation Response*, Dr. Benson makes the point that people who are not religious have some sort of belief system that serves the same purpose. Everyone believes in something. Many have simply never taken the time to think about it.

Open up to the possibility that there is something beyond everyday reality. You might be surprised to discover a long-buried spark of hope inside yourself. Cling to it. That hope is the expression of the survivor inside you. It's the ultimate weapon in your arsenal.

When we are not in touch with the survivor in ourselves, we are likely to fall prey to another strong voice inside of us — the destroyer. This is the voice of negativity, which drags us down into a pit of depression, telling us that there's no hope. It goes on and on like a broken record, saying, "What's the use? You're going to die. You might as well just give up." As soon as I hear that voice, I turn to my *Please God* tapes.

The mind cannot hold positive and negative outlooks at the same time. I make an active choice for the positive.

. . . PERSONAL PERSPECTIVE

ৡ◈

Having had the experience of connecting with my inner survivor, I can use the memory of that experience again and again to reconnect. I can still recall how very close to death I sometimes felt during the long months of chemotherapy. I was a prisoner of my body, trapped in a half-dead container that the medical profession was trying to salvage. I would lie on the couch wondering, "Will I live through these treatments? Can I possibly survive such a murderous ordeal?"

Weak as I was, I found that I was always able to tap into my spiritual high. And no matter what my condition, I would feel at one with myself, with my Creator, with the whole world.

That experience has endured. My life is immeasurably enriched. And this has come about in part because I had cancer. The pain, the suffering, the fear, spurred me on to discover the unending joy of connecting with my purpose. I came to a deeper understanding of the stressful aspects of my life and realized that I could exercise my personal freedom of choice to change them. Perhaps the conditions causing the stress could not be changed, but I could learn to cope with them. As I explored my priorities in life, I could see that most of these stress inducers were tiny, unimportant details.

Having cancer gave me the opportunity to correct a lifetime of unhealthy habits. I learned how my personality fit the cancer profile, rendering me vulnerable to severe illness. While heredity and environment and who knows what other factors certainly contributed their share, my unhealthy habits and repressed, hyperactive personality were bound to take their toll eventually. Cancer gave me the motivation I needed to reform.

Because of these changes, my relationships with my family, my loved ones, and my close friends have improved tremendously. I'm learning how to communicate openly, how to ask for help, how to accept graciously as well as to give. And I am able to open up even more. It's a chain reaction, a continual unfolding to the beauty of life, a beauty I could never wholly appreciate until that life was mortally threatened. The ways of the Lord are indeed mysterious.

It is not my intention to preach to my readers, but as I fought to survive, faith was the strongest weapon in my arsenal. I hope you can, in some form, add it to your own.

Appendix I

COMPREHENSIVE CANCER CENTERS

ALABAMA
Dr. Albert F. LoBuglio,
Director
University of Alabama at
Birmingham Comprehensive
Cancer Center
Basic Health Science Building,
Room 108
1918 University Boulevard
Birmingham, AL 35294
(205) 934-6612

ARIZONA
Dr. Sydney E. Salmon,
Director
University of Arizona Cancer
Center
1501 N. Campbell Avenue
Tucson, AZ 85724
(602) 626-6372

CALIFORNIA
Dr. Brian E. Henderson,
Director
The Kenneth Norris, Jr.,
Comprehensive Cancer Center
University of Southern California
1441 Eastlake Avenue
Los Angeles, CA 90033-0804
(213) 226-2370

Dr. Richard J. Steckel,
Director
Jonsson Comprehensive
Cancer Center
University of California at Los
Angeles (UCLA)
200 Medical Plaza
Los Angeles, CA 90027
(213) 206-0278

CONNECTICUT
Dr. Alan C. Sartorelli, Director
Yale University Comprehensive Cancer Center
333 Cedar Street
New Haven, CT 06510
(203) 785-6338

DISTRICT OF COLUMBIA
Dr. Marc Lippman, Director
Lombardi Cancer Research
Center
Georgetown University
Medical Center
3800 Reservoir Road, N.W.
Washington, D.C. 20007
(202) 687-2192

FLORIDA
Dr. Norman H. Altman,
Director
Sylvester Comprehensive

Cancer Center
University of Miami Medical
School
1475 Northwest 12th Avenue
Miami, FL 33136
(305) 548-4800

MARYLAND
Dr. Albert H. Owens, Jr.,
Center Director
The Johns Hopkins Oncology
Center
600 North Wolfe Street
Baltimore, MD 21205
(301) 955-8638

MASSACHUSETTS
Dr. Baruj Benacerraf,
President
Dana-Farber Cancer Institute
44 Binney Street
Boston, MA 02115
(617) 732-3214

MICHIGAN
Dr. Laurence H. Baker,
Director
Meyer L. Prentis Comprehensive Cancer Center of Metro-
politan Detroit
110 East Warren Avenue
Detroit, MI 48201
(313) 745-4329

Dr. Max Wicha,
Director
University of Michigan Cancer
Center
101 Simpson Drive
Ann Arbor, MI 48109-0752
(313) 936-9583

MINNESOTA
Dr. John S. Kovach, Director
Mayo Comprehensive Cancer
Center
200 First Street Southwest
Rochester, MN 55905

(507) 284-3413

NEW HAMPSHIRE
Dr. O. Ross McIntyre,
Director
Norris Cotton Cancer Center
Dartmouth-Hitchcock Medical
Center
2 Maynard Street
Hanover, NH 03756
(603) 646-5505

NEW YORK
Dr. Paul A. Marks,
President and CEO
Memorial Sloan-Kettering
Cancer Center
1275 York Avenue
New York, NY 10021
1-800-525-2225

Dr. I. Bernard Weinstein,
Director
Columbia University Compre-
hensive Cancer Center
College of Physicians &
Surgeons
630 West 168th Street
New York, NY 10032
(212) 305-6905

Dr. Thomas B. Tomasi,
Director
Roswell Park Cancer Institute
Elm and Carlton Streets
Buffalo, NY 14263
(716) 845-4400

Dr. Vittorio Defendi,
Director
Kaplan Cancer Center
New York University Medical
Center
462 First Avenue
New York, NY 10016-9103
(212) 263-6485

NORTH CAROLINA
Dr. Robert C. Bast, Jr.,
Director
Duke Comprehensive Cancer
Center
P.O. Box 3814
Durham, NC 27710
(919) 286-5515

Dr. Joseph S. Pagano,
Director
Lineberger Comprehensive
Cancer Center
University of North Carolina
School of Medicine
Chapel Hill, NC 27599
(919) 966-4431

Dr. Robert L. Capizzi,
Director
Cancer Center of Wake Forest
University at the Bowman
Gray School of Medicine
300 South Hawthorne Road
Winston-Salem, NC 27103
(919) 748-4354

OHIO
Dr. David E. Schuller,
Director
Ohio State University Compre-
hensive Cancer Center
410 West 10th Avenue
Columbus, OH 43210
(614) 293-8619

PENNSYLVANIA
Dr. Robert C. Young,
President
Fox Chase Cancer Center
7701 Burholme Avenue
Philadelphia, PA 19111
(215) 728-2570

Dr. John H. Glick,
Director
University of Pennsylvania
Cancer Center

3400 Spruce Street
Philadelphia, PA 19104
(215) 662-6364

Dr. Ronald B. Herberman,
Director
Pittsburgh Cancer Institute
200 Meyran Avenue
Pittsburgh, PA 15213-2592
1-800-537-4063

TEXAS
Dr. Charles A. LeMaistre,
President
The University of Texas
M. D. Anderson Cancer Center
1515 Holcombe Boulevard
Houston, TX 77030
(713) 792-3245

VERMONT
Dr. Roger S. Foster, Jr.,
Director
Vermont Cancer Center
University of Vermont
1 South Prospect Street
Burlington, VT 05401
(802) 656-4580

WASHINGTON
Dr. Robert W. Day,
Director
Fred Hutchinson Cancer
Research Center
1124 Columbia Street
Seattle, WA 98104
(206) 467-4675

WISCONSIN
Dr. Paul P. Carbone, Director
Wisconsin Clinical Cancer
Center
University of Wisconsin
600 Highland Avenue
Madison, WI 53792
(608) 263-8090

Appendix II
CLINICAL CANCER CENTERS AND CONSORTIUMS*

CALIFORNIA
Dr. Paul A. Chervenick,
Director
City of Hope National
Medical Center
Beckman Research Institute
1450 East Duarte Road
Duarte, CA 91010
(818) 359-8111, ext. 2292

Dr. Gerard N. Burrow,
Director
University of California at San
Diego Cancer Center
225 Dickinson Street
San Diego, CA 92103
(619) 543-6178

COLORADO
Dr. Paul A. Bunn, Jr.,
Director
University of Colorado Cancer
Center
4200 East Ninth Ave.,
Box B190
Denver, CO 80262
(303) 270-7235

ILLINOIS
Dr. Richard Schilsky,
Director
University of Chicago Cancer
Research Center
5841 South Maryland Avenue
Chicago, IL 60637
(312) 702-9200

NEW YORK
Dr. Matthew D. Scharff,
Director
Albert Einstein College of
Medicine
1300 Morris Park Avenue
Bronx, NY 10461
(212) 920-4826

Dr. Robert A. Cooper, Jr.,
Director
University of Rochester
Cancer Center
601 Elmwood Avenue, Box 704
Rochester, NY 14642
(716) 275-4911

Consortiums* — See page 255.

OHIO
Dr. Nathan A. Berger,
Director
Case Western Reserve
University
University Hospitals of
Cleveland
Ireland Cancer Center
2074 Abington Road
Cleveland, OH 44106
(216) 844-5432

RHODE ISLAND
Dr. Abby Maizel,
Director
Roger Williams Cancer Center
825 Chalkstone Avenue
Providence, RI 02908
(401) 456-2071

TENNESSEE
Dr. Joseph V. Simone,
Director
St. Jude Children's Research
Hospital
332 North Lauderdale Street
Memphis, TN 38101-0318
(901) 522-0306

TEXAS
Dr. Charles A. Coltman, Jr.,
Director
Institute for Cancer Research
and Care
4450 Medical Drive
San Antonio, TX 78229
(512) 616-5580

UTAH
Dr. J. Robert Stewart,
Director
Utah Regional Cancer Center
University of Utah Medical
Center
50 North Medical Drive,
Room 2C10
Salt Lake City, UT 84132
(801) 581-5052

VIRGINIA
Dr. I. David Goldman,
Director
Massey Cancer Center
Medical College of Virginia
Virginia Commonwealth
University
1200 East Broad Street
Richmond, VA 23298
(804) 786-9641

CONSORTIUMS*

ILLINOIS
Dr. Shirley B. Lansky,
Presidcnt and Director
Illinois Cancer Council
  (Consortium)
17th Floor
200 South Michigan Avenue
Chicago, IL 60604
(312) 986-9880

TENNESSEE
Dr. Louis J. Bernard,
Director
Drew Meharry-Morehouse
Consortium Cancer Center
1005 D. B. Todd Boulevard
Nashville, TN 37208
(615) 327-6927

For additional information about cancer, write:
The National Cancer Institute
Office of Cancer Communications
Bethesda, MD 20892
Or call the toll-free telephone number of the Cancer Information Service (CIS) at 1-800-4-CANCER. Spanish-speaking staff members are available to callers.
For publications issued by the National Cancer Institute, call the NCI toll-free telephone number at 1-800-422-6237.

CONSORTIUMS* A consortium is comprised of a network of medical centers and hospitals that participate in clinical trials and experimental treatments.

Appendix III
MAJOR CLINICAL TRIAL
COOPERATIVE GROUPS

Brain Tumor Cooperative Group
Dr. William R. Shapiro,
Chairman
Barrow Neurological Institute
St. Joseph Hospital and
Medical Center
350 West Thomas Road
Phoenix, AZ 85013

Cancer and Leukemia Group B (CALGB)
Dr. Emil Frei, III,
Chairman
Dana-Farber Cancer Institute
44 Binney Street
Boston, MA 02115

Children's Cancer Study Group (CCSG)
Dr. Denman Hammond,
Chairman
University of Southern California
199 North Lake Avenue,
3rd Floor
Pasadena, CA 91101-1859

Eastern Cooperative Oncology Group (ECOG)
Dr. Paul P. Carbone,
Chairman
Wisconsin Clinical Cancer Center
University of Wisconsin
600 Highland Avenue,
Room K4/614
Madison, WI 53792

European Organization for Research on Treatment for Cancer (EORTC)
Dr. Maurice J. Staquet,
Director
Institute Jules Bordet
125 Boulevard de Waterloo
1000 Brussels, Belgium

Gynecologic Oncology Group (GOG)
Dr. Robert C. Park,
Chairman
GOG Headquarters
1234 Market Street,
Suite 1945
Philadelphia, PA 19107

Intergroup Rhabdomyosarcoma Study Group
Dr. Harold M. Maurer, Chairman
Medical College of Virginia
Virginia Commonwealth University
MCV Box 646
Richmond, VA 23298

National Surgical Adjuvant Breast and Bowel Project (NSABP)
Dr. Bernard Fisher, Chairman
University of Pittsburgh
914 Scaife Hall
3550 Terrace Street
Pittsburgh, PA 15261

National Wilms' Tumor Study Group
Dr. Giulio D'Angio, Chairman
Children's Research Center
The Children's Hospital of Philadelphia
3400 Civic Center Boulevard, 9th Floor
Philadelphia, PA 19104

North Central Cancer Treatment Group
Dr. Charles G. Moertel, Chairman
Mayo Clinic
200 First Street, S.W.
Rochester, MN 55905

Pediatric Oncology Group (POG)
Dr. Teresa J. Vietti, Chairman
Del Coronado, Suite 2A
4949 West Pine Street
St. Louis, MO 63108

Radiation Therapy Oncology Group (RTOG)
Dr. James Cox, Chairman
M. D. Anderson Hospital and Tumor Institute
1515 Holcombe Boulevard
Houston, TX 77030

Southwest Oncology Group (SWOG)
Dr. Charles A. Coltman, Chairman
Cancer Therapy and Research Center
4450 Medical Drive
San Antonio, TX 78229

Appendix IV

MULTIDISCIPLINARY SECOND OPINION CENTERS

The following institutions have advised they will when specifically requested provide a multidisciplinary second opinion. The patient *must* specifically make the request. (Arranged by state.)

* indicates free of charge
** indicates that the patient is allowed to sit in front of a pathologist, diagnostic radiologist, surgeon, radiation oncologist, medical oncologist, or other pertinent physicians. They hear their case discussed and are told all their opinions.
# indicates the patient will be interviewed by a physician who will then review the facts with a multidisciplinary panel and relay their comments back to the patient.

A few centers see only those patients with a specific type of cancer, and some limit the number of patients who appear before their panel.

** **Little Rock, AR**
St. Vincent Cancer Center
April Johnson
501-660-3900 *

Tucson, AZ
Arizona Cancer Center
Patty Dalke
602-626-2900

** **San Diego, CA**
University of California,
S.D. Cancer Center
Dr. Mark Green (Dir.),
619-543-6178;
Danny Grady
619-543-3456

** **San Francisco, CA**
Regional Cancer Foundation
Terry Smith
415-775-9956 *

Denver, CO
University of Colorado Cancer
Center
Dr. Paul Bunn, Jr., (Dir.);
Vernie Martin
303-270-7235

New Haven, CT
Yale University
Mary Todd
203-785-6222

 # **Miami, FL
Cedars Medical Center
Marilyn Turner
305-325-5433

** **Iowa City, IA**
Univ. of Iowa Cancer Center
Dr. Peter Jochimsen
319-356-3584

Chicago, IL
Loyola University Medical
Center
Dr. Richard Fisher
708-216-3336

Chicago, IL
Northwestern University
Dr. Leo Gordon
312-908-5284

Detroit, MI
Meyer L. Prentis Comprehensive Cancer Center of Metro-
politan Detroit
Carol Monroe
313-993-0335

** **Kansas City, MO**
R. A. Bloch Cancer Manage-
ment Center
Bobbie Dall (Dir.);
Mobel Goodpasture
816-932-8400 *

** **Hanover, NH**
Norris Cotton Cancer Center
Dr. O. R. McIntyre (Dir.)
603-646-5505

Binghamton, NY
Regional Cancer Center
Lourdes
Dr. Joe Readling (Dir.)
607-798-5431

** **Bronx, NY**
Montefiore Medical Center
Dr. Peter Wiernik (Assoc. Dir.)
212-920-4826

New York, NY
Mount Sinai Cancer Center
Anne Invernale
212-241-6361

Rochester, NY
Univ. of Rochester
Cancer Center
Dori Greene
716-275-4911

Cleveland, OH
Ireland Cancer Center
Joe Gambosi
216-844-5432

Columbus, OH
Arthur G. James Cancer
Hospital and Research Institute
Dr. Bill Farrar
614-293-8890

Philadelphia, PA
Fox Chase Cancer Center
Dr. Paul F. Engstrom
215-728-2986

Philadelphia, PA
University of Pennsylvania
Cancer Center
Florence Allen
215-662-6364;
For breast cancer
patients only:
Karen Bensen-Bilkfist
215-349-5024

** Providence, RI
Roger Williams Cancer Center
Dr. Alan Weitberg
401-456-2581 *

** Knoxville, TN
Thompson Cancer Survival
Center
Nan Shugart
615-541-1757 *

** Memphis, TN
(Children Only)
St. Jude Childrens Hospital
Dr. Joseph Simone
901-522-0301 *

** Galveston, TX
UTMB Cancer Center
Dr. Walter Harvey
409-772-1862

Appendix V

PAIN MANAGEMENT/REFERRAL

American Academy of Pain Management
3600 Sisk Road, Suite 2-D
Modesto, CA 95356
(209) 545-0754

The Academy is involved in research with the academic community and provides comprehensive information on pain management through their publications and conferences for their membership and for other health care professionals as well. Patients can write or call for a referral to a member of the Academy in their vicinity with a specialty in pain management.

American Chronic Pain Association
P.O. Box 850
Rocklin, CA 95677
(916) 632-0922

This is an international Association of over 500 self-help groups in the United States, Canada, New Zealand, Australia, and Russia. They publish a workbook that teaches coping skills and helps individuals to take more responsibility for their own recovery. They stress that groups

work with the medical community and not be used as a substitute for professional services.

American Pain Society
5700 Old Orchard Road
Skokie, IL 60077
(708) 966-5595

An educational and scientific association of clinicians and researchers, the society provides information to the medical profession and other health care professionals about pain medications and pain management through a bimonthly APS Bulletin and an annual scientific meeting.

American Society of Anesthesiologists Committee on Pain Therapy
520 N. Northwest Highway
Park Ridge, IL 60068
(708) 825-5586

Clinical pain therapists can query this Committee for extensive information and guidelines on pain therapy, pain management and other current data. The Committee reports that comprehensive pain management centers are usually directed by a physician (often an anesthesiologist) with a staff of other physicians and health professionals who are experts in pain management. These sophisticated pain units are often found in the departments of anesthesiology in hospitals.

National Chronic Pain Outreach Association (NCPOA)
7979 Old Georgetown Road, Suite 100
Bethesda, MD 20814
(301) 652-4948

This is an information clearing house that provides articles, books, pamphlets, cassettes, and video tapes to those seeking relief from pain and to health care professionals. They publish a quarterly magazine that provides extensive information on coping with pain and pain management. They also sponsor lectures and seminars to increase public awareness. NCPOA provides referrals to chronic pain support groups to health care professionals and medical facilities throughout the United States.

Appendix VI
SUPPORT, INFORMATION AND REFERRAL GROUPS, WISH FULFILLMENT AND SUMMER CAMPS

Support, Information and Referral Groups

American Association for Retired Persons (AARP)
601 E. Street, N.W.
Washington, D.C. 20049
(202) 434-2277

Provides information on living wills, self-help groups and a variety of subjects not limited to topics for the elderly.

American Brain Tumor Association
3725 North Talman Ave.
Chicago, IL 60618
1-800-886-2282 -
Patient Services
(312) 286-5571

Research, treatment and referrals for brain tumor patients.

American Cancer Society (ACS)
National Headquarters:
1599 Clifton Road, N.E.
Atlanta, GA 30329
(404) 320-3333
1-800-227-2345

See the telephone directory for the local chapter.

The ACS offers the following programs:

* CanSurmount — Successfully adjusted cancer patient volunteers provide individual rehabilitation and support to cancer patients.

* I Can Cope — Educational program for cancer patients, families and friends on how to cope effectively with the disease.

* Look Good...Feel Better— Helps cancer patients develop skills to improve their appearance through use of special beauty techniques.

* Laryngectomy Program —

At the request of a physician, cancer patients who have had their voice box removed visit new patients before surgery or after to provide support.

* Ostomy Program — Well-adjusted trained volunteers who have had an ostomy visit patients (before and after surgery) in the hospital to provide moral support and help in learning about care and management.

* Reach to Recovery — Physical and psychological support for mastectomy patients provided by carefully selected and trained, well-adjusted, recovered volunteers.

R. A. Bloch Cancer Management Center
4410 Main Street
Kansas City, MO 64111
(816) 932-8453

Offers educational programs, support groups, brief seminars, and a cancer hot line that matches cancer patients with recovered volunteers.

Cancer Control Society
2043 N. Berendo Street
Los Angeles, CA 90027
(213) 663-7801

Comprehensive information about nontoxic and alternative cancer therapies. Tries to put cancer patients in touch with a patient who has recovered from the same type of cancer.

Cancer Guidance Institute (CGI)
5604 Solway Street
Pittsburgh, PA 15217
(412) 521-2291
Cancer Hot Line:
(412) 782-4023

Associated with the National Coalition for Cancer Survivorship and emphasizes attitude and emotions in the recovery process to help patients cope with the psychological impact of cancer.

Candlelighters Childhood Cancer Foundation
1312 18th Street, N.W.
Washington, D.C. 20036
(202) 659-5136
1-800-366-CCCF

Worldwide affiliated support groups that offer information, emotional support, 24-hour crisis line, transportation and other services for parents of children with cancer.

Children's Hospice International (CHI)
901 N. Washington Street, Suite 700
Alexandria, VA 22314
(703) 684-0330
1-800-24CHILD

A national network that has a database on hospice programs, health care professionals, and support systems. Provides pamphlets and brochures.

The Compassionate Friends
P.O. Box 3696
Oakbrook, IL 60522-3696
(708) 990-0010

A national, nondenominational, self-help, bereavement support organization, with over 635 chapters, for parents, grandparents and siblings.

The Concern for Dying and Educational Counsel
250 West 57th Street
New York, NY 10019

(212) 246-6962
1-800-248-2122

Provides living will forms, including records of patient's treatment wishes, periodic updates on right-to-die legislature and other developments.

Corporate Angel Network, Inc. (CAN)
Building One
Westchester County Airport
White Plains, NY 10604
(914) 328-1313

When space is available, provides transportation via corporate airplanes to treatment centers for cancer patients who do not require special services or assistance to board the plane and one attendant or family member.

ENCORE, YWCA of the U.S.A., National Board
720 Broadway
New York, NY 10003
(212) 614-2700

See telephone directory for local chapter.

Discussion and exercise programs for women who have had breast cancer surgery.

International Association of Cancer Victors
7746 W. Manchester Avenue, Suite 110
Playa del Rey, CA 90293
(213) 306-0748

Over 18 chapters across the U.S. provide a Diagnostic Directory of Alternative Therapies, lists of support groups and patients who have used Alternative Therapies, Newsletters and a journal for members.

Leukemia Society of America (LSA)
733 Third Avenue
New York, NY 10017
(212) 573-8484
1-800-284-4271

Provides information, patient services, including financial aid.

Make Today Count
101½ S. Union Street
Alexandria, VA 22314-3323
(703) 548-9674 or 548-9714

See telephone directory for your local chapter.

Emotional support provided by more than 300 chapters.

National Coalition for Cancer Survivorship
323 Eighth Street, S.W.
Albuquerque, NM 87102
(505) 764-9956

Independent groups and individuals that provide information and resources on support to cancer survivors.

The National Hospice Organization (NHO)
1901 North Moore Street, Suite 901
Arlington, VA 22209
(703) 243-5900

See telephone directory for local program.

Telephone referral service; affiliated groups offer hospice care and guidelines for care of the terminally ill.

National Self-Help Clearing House (NSHC)
25 West 43rd Street, Room 620
New York, NY 10036
(212) 642-2944

Self-help groups clearing house and referral service.

National Women's Health Network (NWHN)

1325 G Street, N.W.
Washington, D.C. 20005
(202) 347-1140

Advocacy program with 300 local groups. Sponsors the Woman's Health Clearing House, a national resource file on all aspects of women's health care.

Peoples Medical Society (PMS)

462 Walnut Street
Allentown, PA 18102
(215) 770-1670

Consumer advocacy program. Also, provides pamphlets of medical rights information and alternative healthcare.

United Ostomy Association (UOA)

36 Executive Park, Suite 120
Irvine, CA 92714
(714) 660-8624

Support and education for ostomy patients.

Y-ME

National Headquarters
18220 Harwood Avenue
Homewood, IL 60430
Hot Line: 1-800-221-2141, 9:00 a.m. to 5:00 p.m. Central Time, Monday through Friday
(708) 799-8228, 24 Hours a Day, Seven Days a Week

Counseling, emotional support and information service for breast cancer patients provided by recovered patients and staff members. They match a patient by age and type of treatment to a volunteer breast cancer patient who may be called at her home. Sponsors affiliates, seminars and workshops all over the country.

Wish Fulfillment

To locate the many wish fulfillment groups for children with life-threatening or chronic illness, check your local telephone directory or call 1-800-4-CANCER. Following are some associations that operate on a nationwide level. They do not limit wishes to the local community.

Brass Ring Society, Inc. (BRS)

314 S. Main Street
Ottawa, KS 66067
(913) 242-1666
1-800-666-9474

Children's Wish Foundation International

8215 Roswell Road, Building 200, Suite 100
Atlanta, GA 30350
1-800-323-9474

Make-A-Wish Foundation of America (National Office)

2600 N. Central Avenue, Suite 936
Phoenix, AZ 85004
(602) 240-6600
1-800-722-WISH

Operation Liftoff

c/o Ernest Bischoff
1171 Kings Avenue
Ben Salem, PA 19020
(215) 639-1586

Starlight Foundation

12233 West Olympic Blvd., Suite 322
Los Angeles, CA 90064
1-800-274-7827

Camps

The camps for children with cancer and other related diseases are too numerous to list. Most of these may be accessed by one call to the CIS (1-800-4-CAN-CER). You also can check your local chapter of the ACS. Many divisions sponsor camp programs throughout the country, or write to Ronald McDonald Children's Charities (RMCC), P.O. Box 11189, Chicago, IL 60611, for a National Directory of Children's Cancer Camps. Following are a few camps that accept campers from throughout the United States, have physicians available 24 hours, are free of charge, and have some unique aspects.

Camp Simcha
c/o Chai Lifeline
National Office
48 West 25th Street
New York, NY 10010
(212) 255-1160

Camp Simcha offers a kosher summer camp program in a traditional setting to children from throughout the world ages 6-16 with cancer or blood-related diseases. Siblings are welcome as well. They have one three-week session, but with the purchase of a permanent facility in Glen Spey in the Catskill Mountains in New York, it is expected that the camp program will be extended. A helicopter is on the premises 24 hours to meet any medical emergencies. Campers return home with a variety of gifts made available by the Chai Lifeline Wish Foundation, and they are offered the opportunity for a five-day trip during the winter season to visit several attractions in Orlando, Florida.

Camp Star Trails
University of Texas
M. D. Anderson Hospital and Tumor Institute
1515 Holcomb
Houston, TX 77030
(713) 792-2465

The camp accepts children ages 5-14 with cancer or any related disease. The camp program includes siblings of campers as well as children with AIDS. They have two one-week sessions during the third and fourth weeks of June. A counselor-in-training program is available for campers. The contact person is Jan Johnson.

Point Sebego Camp Sunshine
RR #1, Box 712
Casco, Maine 04015
(207) 655-3371

This is a family-oriented camp that accepts children with cancer from infancy to 19 years. They are encouraged to come with the entire family unit, if possible. The camp has two one-week sessions in June and two one-week sessions in September. During the fourth session, at the end of September, children with kidney disease and cystic fibrosis are included in the program. Applications are available from medical centers throughout the country that arrange the camp referrals. To locate the center closest to you, contact Nancy Hibbard.

**The Hole-In-The-Wall-Gang
Camp (THITWGC)**
Executive Office
555 Long Wharf Drive
New Haven, CT 06511
(203) 772-0522

The camp has its own beautiful facilities in Ashford near the North Eastern Hills in Storrs, Connecticut. They accept children ages 7-15 with cancer or blood-related diseases from abroad as well as the United States. There are four two-week sessions plus a seven-day session for children with sickle cell anemia, a seven-day session for children who are HIV positive, and a special program at the end of the camp season for siblings. They offer ex-campers a counselor-in-training program. The camp reports they can accommodate kosher or any other special dietary needs of campers.

GLOSSARY

allogeneic: bone marrow transplant technique involving a healthy donor's cells; bone marrow donor and recipient are not genetically identical.

assay: test used to measure something.

autologous: bone marrow transplant technique involving the patient's own cells.

BBB (blood brain barrier): lining of the capillaries in the brain that controls which substances enter and which are prevented from entering.

benign: noncancerous tumor that has a favorable chance for recovery except those found in the brain, which can cause serious side effects.

biopsy: removal of a small piece of tissue from the patient. The tissue sample is then examined under a microscope. A biopsy provides the most reliable basis for diagnosis of cancer.

clinical trials: studies that test new drugs or therapies on human volunteers.

CT scan (or CAT scan): computerized tomography is the use of high speed computer processing combined with X-rays to produce a three-dimensional image of the inside of body. One of the advantages of these scans is that they are noninvasive and do not require the use of contrast dyes, though sometimes a special dye may be injected into the patient's vein to help make abnormal tissue more evident.

DNA (deoxyribonucleic acid): material making up the genes, which takes the form of two spiraling strands. DNA makes up the genetic program of each cell; it is like a foreman who controls the cells' activities.

endorphin: a pain-killing substance produced by the brain that simulates the effects of morphine. It appears to stimulate white cell production or "killer cells" in the immune system.

external beam radiation: a technique by which high doses of X-rays or gamma rays are directed to a patient's tumor by means of a machine.

flow cytometry: technique used to study cells; large numbers of cells are examined very rapidly and the results analyzed by computer.

Hodgkin's disease: a lymphoma that differs from others in that it spreads step-by-step from a given lymph node to neighboring lymph node regions. The disease appears mainly in the young (under age 30) and for 80% of Hodgkin's disease patients a cure is possible.

immune system: the body's defense mechanism; protects against disease by use of "killer white" cells, antibody-producing lymphocytes.

immunotherapy: a boosting of the immune system through vaccines or stimulants to activate the production of antibodies from "killer white" cells which then increase in numbers to eliminate cancer cells.

interleukin-2 (IL-2): substance found in the body used to stimulate the production of immune system cells (lymphokine-activated killer/LAK cells) to fight against cancer cells.

internal radiation: radioactive materials are placed directly into or on the area to be treated; provided by way of a sealed container which is inserted into the body, given orally, or injected.

interstitial radiation: malignant tissues are implanted with and surrounded by needles that contain bits of radioactive isotopes. It is a short-term measure, three to five days, and then removed. A second type involves radioactive material which is permanently implanted directly into the affected organ, and the radiation is released over a period of weeks or months.

intraoperative radiation: radiation delivered directly to the site of a tumor, while a patient is on the operating table and the tumor is exposed. This allows for higher doses to be directed to the tumor.

leukemia: cancer of the blood-forming organs, bone marrow, lymph nodes or spleen, which shows up as an extreme overproduction of white blood cells.

linear accelerators: machines that speed electrons to high energies to produce high voltages of radiation necessary to destroy tumor tissue.

lumpectomy: removal of a malignant lump or small mass from the breast; generally followed by radiation treatment and/or hormonal treatment and chemotherapy.

lymphokine-activated killer (LAK) cells: white-blood-cell derivatives produced by the action of interleukin-2 (IL-2); used to attack cancer cells.

lymphoma: A non-Hodgkin's malignant lymphoma originating in lymphocytes, a type of white blood cell in the lymphoid component of the immune system. Lymphomas usually involve many lymph nodes when they first appear and are seen mostly in people over age 40.

malignant: cancerous. By definition, cancer cells divide too rapidly, are physically different from normal cells, do not function normally and are capable of spreading.

malignant melanoma: the most serious type of skin cancer. If diagnosed early, it is easy to treat; undiagnosed, it spreads rapidly and is difficult to control.

mammogram: a diagnostic procedure for the early detection of breast cancer. A baseline mammogram is recommended for women between the ages of 35 and 40. A yearly mammogram is recommended for women over 50.

mastectomy: surgical removal of the breast and associated lymph nodes.

metastasize (metastatic): the spreading of cancer. Cells from the original tumor travel via the circulatory or lymphatic systems and invade other organs.

methotrexate: a major chemotherapy drug used to treat certain leukemias, lymphomas and sarcomas, breast, brain, and other cancers.

modalities: methods.

monoclonal antibodies: antibodies "trained" to locate or attack a target mass of cells; used in cancer detection, diagnosis and treatment.

MRI (magnetic resonance imaging): a highly detailed diagnostic device that portrays the body's soft, internal tissues.

multidisciplinary: involving more than one area of expertise.

oncologist: a physician who specializes in treating tumors and cancer.

palliative treatment: treating the symptoms without affecting a cure, such as treatment to relieve pain.

palpable: readily felt by the hands during physical examination.

pathologist: a physician who interprets blood tests and tissue specimens to ascertain the origin and progression of disease.

PDQ (Physicians' Data Query): a computerized information service providing immediate access to the latest cancer research; offered through NCI, or a search can be requested from the CIS nearest to you.

pharmacologist: an expert on drugs.

prognosis: how an illness or disease is expected to progress.

protocol: the standards or detailed plan by which experimental or established treatments are executed.

psychoneuroimmunology (PNI): a new field of medicine devoted to the study of the mind-body connection through the study of the interrelationship of the mind, the nervous system, and the immune system.

radiation oncologist or radiation therapist: a physician with a specialty in the use of radiation to treat disease who prescribes and directs the course of radiation treatment.

solid tumors: tumors which form a mass or growth, such as those of the breast, ovaries, bladder, colon and prostate and certain cancers of the lung.

tamoxifen (Nolvadex): antiestrogen drug that blocks the growth-promoting effects of estrogen in estrogen-dependent tumors, such as breast tumors.

toxicologist: expert on substances that are harmful to the body.

tumor markers: chemical substances produced by a tumor as it grows. Different kinds of tumors produce different substances, and so analyzing these substances can tell physicians certain things about the location and nature of the growth.

white cells (leukocytes): made in the bone marrow, cells that help fight fungal and bacterial infections. They can capture, destroy and remove germs from the body.

BIBLIOGRAPHY

Achterberg, Jeanne. *Imagery In Healing: Shamanism And Modern Medicine.* Boston: New Science Library, 1985.

Aihara, Herman. *Acid & Alkaline.* Oroville, CA: The George Ohsawa Macrobiotic Foundation, 1980.

Airola, Paavo. *Are You Confused?* Phoenix: Health Plus, Publishers, 1971.

_____. *Cancer Causes, Prevention & Treatment: The Total Approach.* Phoenix: Health Plus, Publishers, 1972.

Alexander, Franz, M.D. *Psychosomatic Medicine.* New York: W. W. Norton, 1950.

Allison, Malory E. "Cancer Biology: Targeting The Supply Lines." *The Harvard Mental Health Letter*, Vol. 16, No. 7 (May, 1991), pp. 2-4.

Barber, Joseph, Ph.D., and Jean Gitelson. "Cancer Pain Psychological Management Using Hypnosis." *CA — A Cancer Journal for Clinicians*, Vol. 30, No. 3 (May/June, 1980), pp. 130-136.

Benjamin, Harold H., Ph.D., with Richard Trubo. *From Victim to Victor -- The Wellness Community Guide to Fighting for Recovery for Cancer Patients and Their Families.* Los Angeles: Jeremy P. Tarcher, Inc., 1987.

Benkendorf, Jayne. *The Food Bible.* Highland City, FL: Rainbow Books, Inc., 1991.

Benson, Herbert, M.D., with William Proctor. *Beyond the Relaxation Response: How to Harness the Healing Power of Your Personal Beliefs.* New York: Times Books, 1984.

_____., with Miriam Z. Klipper. *The Relaxation Response.* New York: Avon Books, 1976.

Berger, Stuart. *Dr. Berger's Immune Power Diet.* New York: New American Library, 1985.

Bland, Jeffrey. *Digestive Enzymes.* New Canaan, CT: Keats Publishing, Inc., 1983.

Bloch, Richard, and Annette Bloch. *Cancer . . . There's Hope.* Kansas City, MO: Cancer Connection, Inc., 1981.

Bok, Derek. "Needed: A New Way to Train Doctors." *Harvard Magazine*, Vol. 86, No. 5 (May/June, 1984), pp. 32-43.

Boly, William. "Cancer, Inc." *Hippocrates*, Vol. 3, No. 1 (January/February, 1989), pp. 38-52.

Borysenko, Joan, with Larry

Rothstein. *Minding the Body, Mending the Mind.* Reading, MA: Addison-Wesley, 1987.

Bruning, Nancy. *Coping with Chemotherapy.* Garden City, NY: Dial Press/Doubleday, 1985.

Caplan, Brina. "Kiyo Morimoto and the Art of Inclusion." *Harvard Magazine,* Vol. 88, No. 2 (November/December, 1985), pp. 79-82.

Castleman, Michael. "Doctors Are Mistreating Cancer — A Shocking Report." *Redbook,* (January, 1990), p. 98.

Chang, Jeff, and Bryan Hiebert. "Relaxation Procedures with Children: A Review." *Medical Psychotherapy: An International Journal,* Yearbook, Vol. 2 (1989), pp. 163-176.

Clark, Matt. "A President's Cancer Scare." *Newsweek,* (July 22, 1985), p. 14.

Cochran, Joan. "Flow Cytometry: Revealing the Cell's Secrets." *Cedars Now!,* Vol. 2, No. 1 (1989), p. 3-4.

Copeland, M. Edward, III, M.D. "Intravenous Hyperalimentation as an Adjunct to Cancer Patient Management." *The Cancer Bulletin,* No. 30 (1978), pp. 102-108.

Cousins, Norman. *Anatomy of an Illness.* New York: Bantam Books, 1981.

_____. *Head First — The Biology of Hope.* New York: Dutton, 1989.

Craig, Jean. *Between Hello & Goodbye.* Los Angeles: Jeremy P. Tarcher, Inc. 1991.

Dana-Farber Cancer Institute. "Scientists Pioneer New Approach to Cancer Treatment.", ed. Hallie Baron.

Centerline, Vol. 14, No. 5 (September, 1988), p. 12.

DeVita, Vincent T., M.D. *Cancer Treatment.* Bethesda, MD: National Institute of Health No. 84-1807, 1987.

_____. "Why More People Are Surviving Cancer." *U.S. News and World Report,* Vol. 93, No. 12 (September 20, 1982), pp. 72-74.

Diffily, Anne. "Americans and 'The Big C'." *Brown Alumni Monthly,* Vol. 88, No. 3 (November, 1987), pp. 30-34.

Eysenck, Hans J. "Health's Character." *Psychology Today,* Vol. 22, No. 12 (December, 1988), pp. 28-35.

Fay, Martha. *A Mortal Condition: A New Look at Living with Cancer.* New York: Berkley Books, 1983.

Fink, John M. *Third Opinion.* Garden City Park, NY: Avery Publishing Group, Inc., 1988.

Fiore, Neil A. Ph.D. *Road Back to Health: Coping with the Emotional Side of Cancer.* New York: Bantam Books, 1984.

Frankl, Viktor, M.D. *Man's Search for Meaning.* New York: Pocket Books, 1980.

Gallagher, Winifred. "Mind/Body Therapy: The Healing Touch." *American Health,* Vol. III, No. 8 (October, 1988), p. 45.

Gelman, David, et al. "Depression." *Newsweek,* (May 4, 1987), p. 48.

_____. "The Mind-Body Connection." *Newsweek,* (November 7, 1988), p. 88.

Glassman, Judith. *The Cancer Survivors: And How They Did It.* New York: Doubleday,

1983.

Glucksberg, Harold, M.D., and Jack W. Singer, M.D. *Cancer Care, A Personal Guide.* Baltimore: Johns Hopkins University Press, 1980.

Gold, Michael. *A Conspiracy of Cells.* Albany, NY: State of New York Press, 1986.

Gray, Robert. *The Colon Health Handbook*, 10th ed. Reno: Emerald Publishing, 1985.

Griffin, G. Edward. *World Without Cancer: The Story of Vitamin B-17.* Westlake Village, CA: American Media, 1974.

Gunther, John. *Death Be Not Proud.* New York: Harper & Row, Publishers, 1949.

Hinds, Katherine. "Stephanie LaFarge: Riding Piggyback Into Death." *Brown Alumni Monthly*, Vol. 84, No. 2 (October, 1983), pp. 22-27.

Hoffmann, Stephen, M.D. "When the Patient Knows Best." *American Health*, Vol. VII, No. 10 (December, 1988), p. 79.

Holland, Jimmie C., M.D. "Understanding the Cancer Patient." *CA — A Cancer Journal for Clinicians*, Vol. 30, No. 2 (March/April, 1980), pp. 103-112.

Holland, Jimmie C., Ann Hughes Korzun, Susan Tross, Peter Silverfarb, Michael Perry, Robert Comis, and Martin Oster. "Pancreatic Cancer and Depression." *The Harvard Medical School Mental Health Letter*, Vol. 3, No. 8 (February, 1987), p. 7.

Houck, Catherine. "Psychosomatic Illness: More Than We Imagine." *Cosmopolitan*, (October, 1983).

Jampolsky, Gerald. *Love Is Let-*
ting Go Of Fear. Millbrae, CA: Celestial Arts, 1979.

Kaplan, Aryeh. *Jewish Meditation — A Practical Guide.* New York: Schocken Books, Inc., 1985.

Kaprio, Jaakko, Markku Koskenvuo, and Heli Rita. "Dangers Of Bereavement." *The Harvard Medical School Mental Health Letter*, Vol. 4, No. 5 (November, 1987), pp. 1-4.

Kenneth Norris, Jr., Cancer Hospital and Research Institute Annual Report, 7/1/84-6/30/85. Los Angeles: University of Southern California, 1985.

Kirschmann, John D., and Lavon J. Dunne. *Nutrition Almanac*, 2nd ed. New York: McGraw-Hill Book Company, 1984.

Kohler, Jean Charles, and Mary Alice Kohler. *Healing Miracles from Macrobiotics: A Diet for All Diseases.* West Nyack, NY: Parker Publishing Company, Inc., 1979.

Kübler-Ross, Elisabeth. *Death: The Final Stage of Growth.* Englewood, NJ: Prentice-Hall, 1975.

_____. *On Death and Dying.* New York: Macmillan Publishing Company, Inc., 1969.

Kushi, Michio. *The Cancer Prevention Diet.* New York: St. Martin's Press, 1983.

Lambert, Craig. "The Chopra Prescriptions." *Harvard Magazine*, Vol. 92, No. 1 (September/October, 1989), pp. 23-28.

Lauerman, John. "A Nutritional Block Against Cancer?" *Harvard Magazine*, (May/June, 1987), pp. 40-42.

Lavigne, John V., Ph.D., and

Michael Ryan. "Psychologic Adjustment of Siblings of Children with Chronic Illness." *Pediatrics*, Vol. 63, No. 4 (April, 1979), pp. 616-626.

Lawrence, Walter, Jr., M.D. "Improving Cancer Treatment by Expanding Clinical Trials." *Oncology Times*, Vol. XI, No. 5 (May, 1989), p. 2.

Lazarus, Hillard M., M.D. "Extended Study of Bone Marrow Transplantation at the Ireland Cancer Center." *Oncology On-Line*, Vol. 2, No. 5 (September-October, 1986), p. 1.

LeShan, Lawrence L., Ph.D. *You Can Fight for Your Life: Emotional Factors in the Causation of Cancer.* New York: Evans, 1977.

Locke, Stephen, M.D., and Douglas Colligan. *The Healer Within.* New York: New American Library, 1987.

Long, Ruth Yale, Ph.D. *Crackdown on Cancer with Good Nutrition.* Houston: Nutrition Education Association, Inc., 1983.

Maher, Thomas M., and Malcolm Schwartz, M.D. *A Doctor Discusses Cancer.* Chicago: Budlong Press, 1981.

Markel, William M., and Virginia B. Sinon. *The Hospice Concept.* American Cancer Society Professional Education Publication, 1978.

Mayo Foundation. "Cancer Prevention." *HealthTalk*, Vol. 11 (Winter, 1988).

Mendelsohn, Robert S., M.D. *Confessions of a Medical Heretic.* New York: Warner Books, 1979.

_____. *Male Practice — How Doctors Manipulate Women.* Chicago: Contemporary Books, Inc., 1981.

Mills, Joan. "Breakdown! A Journey Through Stress." *Reader's Digest*, (January, 1982), pp. 49-53.

Mindel, Earl. *Vitamin Bible.* New York: Warner Books, 1981.

Monagan, David. "Fatal Emotions." *Reader's Digest*, Vol. 128 (May, 1986), pp. 123-126.

Morra, Marion, and Eve Potts. *Choices: Realistic Alternatives in Cancer Treatment,* rev. ed. New York: Avon Books, 1987.

_____. *Understanding Your Immune System.* New York: Avon Books, 1986.

Nash, David T. *Medical Mayhem.* New York: Walker and Company, 1985.

National Cancer Institute. *Division of Cancer Treatment 1987 Annual Report.* Bethesda, MD: U.S. Department of Health and Human Services, 1987.

_____. *1987 Annual Cancer Statistics Review.* Bethesda, MD: U.S. Department of Health and Human Services, 1988.

National Institute of Health. *Research Advances and Opportunities in the Biomedical Sciences.* Bethesda, MD: U.S. Department of Health and Human Services, 1987.

Nauts, Helen Coley. *Breast Cancer: Immunological Factors Affecting Incidence, Prognosis and Survival,* Monograph #18. New York: Cancer Research Institute, Inc., 1984.

Northern California Cancer Program Annual Report,

July, 1983-June 30, 1984. Palo Alto, CA, 1984.

Noyes, Diana Doan, and Peggy Mellody, R.N. *Beauty and Cancer.* Los Angeles: AC Press, 1988.

"Nutrition News," ed. Robert Rodale. *Prevention,* (June, 1989), p. 20.

Passwater, Richard A. *Cancer and Its Natural Therapies.* New Canaan, CT: Keats Publishing, Inc., 1983.

Persky, Victoria W., Joan Kempthorne-Rawson, and Richard B. Shekelle. "Depression And Cancer." *The Harvard Medical School Mental Health Letter,* Vol. 4, No. 9 (March, 1988), p. 7.

Podolsky, Doug M. "Breast Cancer and the Pill." *American Health.* (April, 1989), p. 18.

Radmacher, Sally, and Charles Sheridan. "The Global Inventory of Stress: A Comprehensive Approach to Stress Management." *Medical Psychotherapy; An International Journal,* Yearbook, Vol. 2 (1989), pp. 183-188.

Radner, Gilda. *It's Always Something.* New York: Simon and Schuster, 1989.

Revici, Emanuel, M.D. *Research in Physiopathology as Basis of Guided Chemotherapy.* New York: Van Nostrand Company, Inc., 1961.

Rohé, Fred. *Metabolic Ecology: A Way to Win the Cancer War.* Winfield, KS: Wedgestone Press, 1982.

Rollin, Betty. *Last Wish.* New York: Linden Press, 1985.

Rosenfeld, Isadore, M.D. *Second Opinion: Your Medical Alternatives.* New York: Linden Press, 1981.

Ross, Walter S. "At Last, An Anti-Cancer Diet." *Reader's Digest,* (February, 1983), pp. 78-82.

Rotman, Boris. "Which Cancer Drugs Are Right for What Patient?" *Brown Alumni Monthly,* Vol. 84, No. 5 (February, 1984), pp. 52-53.

St. Jude Children's Research Hospital. *85-86 Scientific Report, No. 24.* Memphis, 1986.

Salmon, Sydney E. "Chemosensitivity Testing: Another Chapter." *Journal of the National Cancer Institute,* (1990), pp. 82-83 (editorial).

Satir, Virginia M. *Peoplemaking.* Palo Alto, CA: Science and Behavior Books, 1972.

Sattilaro, Anthony J., M.D. *Recalled by Life: The Story of My Recovery from Cancer.* Boston: Houghton Mifflin Company, 1982.

Scharffenberg, J. A., M.D., M.P.H. "What You Can Do to Cut Your Cancer Risk." *Life & Health,* Special Issue (1979), pp. 18-21.

Schur, Rabbi Tsvi G. *Illness and Crisis: Coping the Jewish Way.* New York: National Conference of Synagogue Youth/Union of Orthodox Jewish Congregations, 1987.

Segell, Michael. "Doctor Fear." *American Health,* (September, 1989), p. 83.

Seliger, Susan. "Stress Can Be Good for You." *New York,* (August 2, 1982), pp. 20-24.

Sellick, Scott, and George Fitzsimmons. "Biofeedback: An Exercise in Self-Efficacy." *Medical Psychotherapy: An*

International Journal, Yearbook, Vol. 2 (1989), pp. 115-124.

Sevin, B. U., Z. L. Peng, J. P. Perras, P. Ganjei, M. Penalver, and H. E. Averette. "Application of an ATP-bioluminescence Assay in Human Tumor Chemosensitivity Testing." *Gynecologic Oncology,* No. 31 (1988), pp. 191-204.

Seyle, Hans. *The Stress of Life.* New York: McGraw-Hill, 1978.

Shils, Maurice E., M.D., Sc.D. "Enteral Nutritional Management of the Cancer Patient." *The Cancer Bulletin,* No. 30 (1978), pp. 98-101.

Shimkin, Michael B., M.D. *Science & Cancer,* 4th ed. Bethesda, MD: U.S. Department of Health and Human Services, 1983.

Siegel, Bernie S., M.D. *Love, Medicine & Miracles.* New York: Harper & Row, 1986.

Sim, M. K., and J. K. Grewal. "Chinese Diaphragmatic Breathing as an Adjunct to Relaxation: Effects on EEG." *Medical Psychotherapy: An International Journal,* Yearbook, Vol. 2 (1989), pp. 157-162.

Simonton, O. Carl, M.D., Stephanie Matthews-Simonton, and James L. Creighton. *Getting Well Again.* New York: Bantam Books, 1981.

Smith, Eleanor. "Fighting Cancerous Feelings." *Psychology Today,* Vol. 22, No. 5 (May, 1988), pp. 22-23.

Solzhenitsyn, Aleksandr. *Cancer Ward.* trans. Nicholas Bethell and David Burg. New York: Bantam Books, 1969.

Sontag, Susan. *Illness as Metaphor.* New York: Vintage Books, 1978.

Spiegel, David, M.D. "Psychosocial Treatment And Cancer Survival." *The Harvard Medical School Mental Health Letter,* Vol. 7, No. 7 (January, 1991), p. 4-6.

Thomas, Lewis, M.D. "Cancer Risk: Less Than We Fear." *Reader's Digest,* Vol. 124 (February, 1984), pp. 142-143.

Times of Challenge. ed. Seryl Sander. Brooklyn: Mesorah Publications, Ltd., 1988.

Tropp, Jack. *Cancer: A Healing Crisis.* Los Angeles: Cancer Resource Center, 1980.

University of Wisconsin Clinical Cancer Center. *Annual Report 1986.* Madison, WI: 1986.

van Eys, Jan, Ph.D., M.D. "Nutrition and Cancer in Children." *The Cancer Bulletin,* No. 30 (1978), pp. 93-97.

Von Hoff, Daniel D. "He's not going to talk about *in vitro* predictive assays again, is he?" *Journal of the National Cancer Institute,* No. 82 (1990), pp. 96-101.

Weiner, Richard. "Orienting Patients with Chronic Pain." *Medical Psychotherapy: An International Journal,* Yearbook, Vol. 2 (1989), pp. 49-52.

Woltering, Eugene A. "Tumor Chemosensitivity Testing: An Evolving Technique." *Laboratory Medicine,* No. 21 (1990), pp. 82-84.

Wunderlich, Ray C., Jr., M.D., and Dwight K. Kalita. *Candida Albicans.* New Canaan, CT: Keats Publishing, Inc., 1984.

INDEX

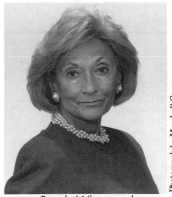

Photograph by Marshall Gross

Sarah Winograd

ABOUT THE AUTHOR

Sarah Winograd graduated from the University of Rhode Island, *summa cum laude*, with a B. A. in Psychology. She went on to earn her M.S. degree in Community Counseling from Barry University, Miami, Florida.

A Fellow and Diplomate of the American Board of Medical Psychotherapists, she is also certified by the National Board of Certified Counselors and licensed as a Mental Health Counselor by the State of Florida.

During her professional career, Mrs. Winograd has developed a program for training health care professionals and recovered cancer patients to counsel cancer patients and their families. Currently she serves as a Cancer Consultant to non-profit organizations in Massachusetts, New York, California and Florida and is a member of the Institutional Review Board of Guidelines, Inc., Miami, Florida. She also serves as Coordinator of the Women's Cancer Recovery Program of The Family Workshop of the Miami Beach Community Hospital (formerly St. Francis Hospital) and The Center for Psychological Growth in Miami and as Director of Mental Health and Social Services of the Jewish Outreach Project of Greater Miami, Inc., in Florida, while maintaining her private practice as a psychotherapist in Miami Beach, Florida.

Mrs. Winograd has spoken extensively on cancer prevention and care, and marital and family relations. She is listed in *Who's Who Among Human Services Professionals* and *The National Distinguished Service Register*.

Dear Reader:

Any information, concerning innovative cancer therapies that you might like to share with the author, will be welcome. Your insights could be beneficial to others.

Please mail your comments and information to . . .

Sarah Winograd
c/o Rainbow Books, Inc.
P. O. Box 430
Highland City, FL 33846

ORDER FORM

GET HELP, GET POSITIVE, GET WELL

For additional copies of *Get Help, Get Positive, Get Well*, telephone TOLL FREE 1-800-356-9315. MasterCard/VISA accepted.

To order *Get Help, Get Positive, Get Well* direct from the publisher, send your check or money order to Rainbow Books, Inc., Order Dept., P.O. Box 430, Highland City, FL 33846-0430.
Trade Softcover — $16.95 plus $3.00 shipping and handling ($19.95 postpaid).

For QUANTITY PURCHASES, telephone Rainbow Books, Inc. (813) 648-4420 or write to the publisher, Rainbow Books, Inc., P.O. Box 430, Highland City, FL 33846-0430.